IMAGES
of America

THE BABIES HOSPITAL OF NEW YORK

ON THE COVER: Patients and their parents wait expectantly for Christmas festivities to begin at Babies Hospital in December 1926. The location is the second hospital building (1902–1929) at the corner of Lexington Avenue and East Fifty-Fifth Street. The hospital's 1926 annual report noted that the celebration featured not only toys for children and a towering Christmas tree but also "bundles of warm clothing for the many who needed that kind of help." (Archives & Special Collections, Augustus C. Long Health Sciences Library, Columbia University Irving Medical Center.)

IMAGES
of America

THE BABIES HOSPITAL OF NEW YORK

Michael Weiner, MD, and Stephen E. Novak
Foreword by Jordan S. Orange, MD, PhD

ARCADIA
PUBLISHING

ISBN 978-1-4671-0737-2

Published by Arcadia Publishing
Charleston, South Carolina

Printed in the United States of America

Library of Congress Control Number: 2021948148

For all general information, please contact Arcadia Publishing:
Telephone 843-853-2070
Fax 843-853-0044
E-mail sales@arcadiapublishing.com
For customer service and orders:
Toll-Free 1-888-313-2665

Visit us on the Internet at www.arcadiapublishing.com

The Babies Hospital of New York *is dedicated to the physicians, scientists, nurses, health care providers, patients, and families who have walked through the hallowed doors of the institution and made it great. The past is the bedrock from which the present is reached, and the present provides the path forward for the future.*

Contents

FOREWORD

The Babies Hospital of New York is a profound institution with an extraordinary legacy. Founded by five inspiring women over 130 years ago, their stories and vision set the institution on a path to excellence in care and innovation for children and in medicine in general. So many relevant firsts in pediatrics derive from work done at and ideas originating from the Babies Hospital. The discovery of many diseases, diagnostics, and treatments, as well as the training of so many leaders and visionaries in children's health, are part of the history of the hospital. Although the institution now bears a different name, the legacy of Babies stands strong and is a story worth telling. As the chair of the Department of Pediatrics at Columbia University and the physician in chief of the Children's Hospital, which traces back to Babies Hospital, I have had the privilege of learning of its contributions and past. I have reviewed annual reports dating back to the very beginning, many of which have been digitized and are publicly available on the website of the Long Library Archives & Special Collections. If there is one thing that has from my perspective always been present, it is a deep sense of mission, which from its inception was to relieve "mental and physical distress" and to never refuse a patient even if prospects were considered "hopeless." This has resulted in an institution and community of tremendous courage, commitment, camaraderie, and heart. I thank you for taking the time to learn about the Babies Hospital through the collected, preserved images and vignettes assembled on these pages. I hope the profound mission and heart emerge as they both remain relevant, palpable, inspiring, and vibrant to this day.

—Jordan Orange, MD, PhD
Reuben S. Carpentier Professor of Pediatrics; chair, Department of Pediatrics,
Columbia University Irving Medical Center

ACKNOWLEDGMENTS

Great academic medical centers and hospitals are composed of health care providers, physicians, nurses, learners, philanthropists, courageous children, parents, and families. The Babies Hospital is such an institution, replete with historical richness, innovation, discovery, and important medical firsts. Founded in a brownstone on the east side of Manhattan in 1887 by sisters, Drs. Sarah and Julia McNutt, the Babies Hospital was the first hospital in New York City and the fourth oldest in the United States exclusively for children. The legacy of the hospital was advanced by L. Emmett Holt, MD, the first chair of the Department of Pediatrics, scholar, mentor, and author of *Holt's Diseases of Infancy and Childhood*. Holt's later successor, Rustin McIntosh, created subspecialty services in hematology-oncology, radiology, and neurology among others during his almost-30-year tenure.

The inspiration for *The Babies Hospital of New York* is Jordan S. Orange, MD, PhD, the Reuben S. Carpentier Professor; chair of the Department of Pediatrics, Columbia University Vagelos College of Physicians and Surgeons; and pediatrician in-chief of NewYork-Presbyterian Morgan Stanley Children's Hospital. His penchant for history and belief that our future is rooted in our past made this book possible.

Unless otherwise noted, all images appear courtesy of Archives & Special Collections of the Augustus C. Long Health Sciences Library, Columbia University Irving Medical Center.

Members of the NewYork-Presbyterian Hospital development office and special events team of the Morgan Stanley Children's Hospital also provided photographs.

Royalties from *The Babies Hospital of New York* will be donated to Columbia Children's Health.

—Michael Weiner, MD

—Stephen E. Novak, head of Archives & Special Collections,
A.C. Long Health Sciences Library

INTRODUCTION

The history of children's health in New York City dates back to 1767, a total of 120 years before the opening of the Babies Hospital. Dr. Samuel Bard, one of America's first and most prominent early physicians, incorporated pediatrics as part of King's College, which became Columbia University. Bard wrote the first American textbook on obstetrics and pediatrics, describing "blue babies" and the diseases of infants in the first year of life and the first definitive description of diphtheria. Bard's distinguished career was capped when he was appointed the first dean of medicine at the Columbia University College of Physicians and Surgeons.

The mid-19th century was influenced by Tammany Hall, an institution that dominated New York City during this era. Reforms instituted by Mayor Fernando Wood, the first Tammany Hall politician to hold the office, led to police riots, gangs, and violence. The country was consumed by the Civil War; the city provided a major source of troops, supplies, equipment, and financing for the Union army, and the powerful elite politicians and newspaper editors helped shape public opinion in favor of the policies of Pres. Abraham Lincoln.

The post–Civil War period ushered in an age that laid the foundation of many of New York's preeminent cultural institutions, the Metropolitan Museum of Art, the Metropolitan Opera, and the American Museum of Natural History. The Statue of Liberty welcomed a flood of European immigration from Germany, Italy, Ireland, and Eastern Europe who entered New York harbor first through Castle Clinton and then Ellis Island, which opened in 1892. European immigration brought further social upheaval, and Old World criminal societies rapidly exploited the already corrupt municipal machine politics of Tammany Hall. Housing, especially in the southern tip of Manhattan, became crowded with newly built tenements and flimsy shacks. Italians settled around Mulberry Street, an area later to be known as Little Italy, whereas Yiddish-speaking East European Jews populated the Lower East Side.

The first New York City Department of Health was created in 1870 by Tammany Hall boss William Tweed, head of the Democratic Party; he appointed Charles Chandler, PhD, a professor of chemistry at Columbia University, as the first commissioner of health in 1873. Dr. Chandler instituted a milk inspection program, directed a chemical laboratory that examined water, milk, and food supplies, and inaugurated programs to combat rampant epidemics of cholera, typhus, anthrax, and tuberculosis.

In the 1880s, Robert Koch and Louis Pasteur developed and popularized the germ theory that led to a new diphtheria antitoxin. Armed with this new vaccine, health commissioner Dr. Herman Biggs opened the city's first bacteriology lab and directed a citywide free program to inoculate the poor against diphtheria.

Against a background of corruption, immigration, poverty, and rampant infectious diseases, Dr. Sarah McNutt and her sister Dr. Julia McNutt incorporated the Babies Hospital, the first hospital exclusively for sick children less than two years of age in New York City and the fourth oldest in the United States, in November 1887. With the financial support of wealthy New Yorkers like

Mrs. William H. Vanderbilt (Maria Louisa), Mrs. Ambrose C. Kingsland (Mary), and Mrs. Abram S. Hewitt (Sarah A.), a four-story brownstone at the northeast corner of Lexington Avenue and Fifty-Fifth Street was purchased for $26,000. The *Real Estate Record & Builders' Guide* described the building as a "handsome dwelling." Nell Nelson in the *Evening World* wrote, "The Babies' Hospital is the only institution of its kind in the country, and only one in the world that is reserved for the exclusive accommodation of babies."

The first year of the Babies Hospital was tumultuous; the fledging hospital had financial, political, and space issues. A neighbor complained "that the hospital was a nuisance in the neighborhood." A local magistrate, Judge Miles Beach, noted that there was a covenant in the deed restricting the property to residential use only and ruled that the hospital must find a new location.

Drs. Sarah and Julia McNutt were not prepared for Judge Beach's legal decision and were obliged to withdraw from the Babies Hospital a year after assisting in founding it. In 1889, Dr. L. Emmett Holt succeeded Sarah McNutt as director and attending physician. He guided the institution for more than 30 years.

Under Holt's leadership, a new building was identified: two four-story houses at 657 and 659 Lexington Avenue at Fifty-Fifth Street, purchased in 1889, were refurbished and opened in 1891. Early on in Holt's tenure at Babies Hospital, he was concerned by the lack of budgetary support from either New York State or City and bemoaned the fact that the hospital was solely dependent on volunteer contributions. Holt was preoccupied with the finances of the Babies Hospital and viewed philanthropy as the path forward. He wrote in 1892, "When we consider the immense mortality among infants under one year of age it is surprising that some of the means which we have been so lavishly used in this city for taking care of sick men and women should not have been appropriated for the care of sick babies."

In 1902, the hospital moved to a modern seven-story building on the corner of Fifty-Fifth Street and Lexington Avenue that doubled the size of the original facility and included outpatient facilities, laboratories, and 70 beds.

Holt was a favored lecturer and teacher at the College of Physicians and Surgeons of Columbia University; he became a professor of pediatrics at the medical school in 1901. His efforts established the foundation of an academic enterprise dedicated to combating infectious diseases, reducing infant mortality, and promoting new specialties such as surgery. Under Holt's guidance, the Babies Hospital became the most celebrated pediatric hospital in the United States and Holt the foremost pediatrician in the country.

As battles raged in Europe during World War I, events in New York City affected the Babies Hospital greatly. First, a major outbreak of polio, which caused paralysis and death in children and adults, reached epidemic proportions in the summer of 1916. Containment efforts were hamstrung by ignorance of how the disease spread, and the epidemic registered 8,991 cases and 2,448 deaths in the city alone. It would go down as the worst polio outbreak in New York history.

Only two years later, the worldwide influenza pandemic, referred to as the Spanish flu, hit New York City. In the Babies Hospital annual report, Holt referred to the illness as "the Black Plague of 1918." The hospital treated 130 total cases of children with influenza, none of whom died.

Herbert Wilcox succeeded L. Emmett Holt as the director of the Babies Hospital and pediatrician-in-chief in 1922. The major accomplishments during his tenure were, first, to expand inpatient and outpatient services and to increase the medical, nursing, and support staff, and second, to facilitate the construction of the new Babies Hospital on the campus of the Columbia-Presbyterian Medical Center. In 1929, the Babies Hospital relocated to a new building on Broadway and West 168th Street.

The new facility expanded to 190 beds and accepted patients to the age of 12. Dr. Rustin McIntosh, a famed pediatrician, became the pediatrician-in-chief in 1931, and during his tenure, the Babies Hospital was among the first in the country to develop programs in neonatal care, pediatric surgery, radiology, neurology, hematology-oncology, and psychiatry. Babies Hospital defined modern pediatrics. Columbia-Presbyterian physicians shed light on many conditions, such as Kasabach-Merritt syndrome, McCune-Albright syndrome, Riley-Day syndrome, and shaken baby syndrome. They also identified the difference between celiac disease and cystic fibrosis, described the sweat test for cystic fibrosis, and created the Apgar score.

Babies Hospital has evolved significantly over the past century. The building was renovated, and the spaces were reconfigured to accommodate programmatic changes and expansion. During World War II, the hospital announced plans to expand and launched a major capital improvement initiative implemented in the early 1960s. In 1968, Babies Hospital South was erected immediately adjacent to the older building, and it opened in the early 1970s, nearly doubling the size of the hospital. The contemporary new building enhanced service to children throughout the metropolitan region. It was said that "If your child was ill the only place to be was the Babies Hospital."

In 1977, Dr. Michael Katz, a celebrated specialist in infectious diseases, became the chair of pediatrics. Columbia doctors performed early pediatric heart transplants, described the syndrome of persistent fetal circulation, and developed continuous positive alveolar pressure (CPAP) for premature infants.

In the late 1990s, a renovation to the pediatric intensive care unit (PICU), sponsored by Morgan Stanley, was followed up by a much larger addition to the hospital, also sponsored and named after the financial firm. In 2004, Dr. John Driscoll, working with colleagues at NewYork-Presbyterian Hospital, opened the present 265,000-square-foot inpatient facility, the NewYork-Presbyterian/Morgan Stanley Children's Hospital. The new facility is the largest and most renowned children's facility in the Tri-State Area and ranks among the top in the nation in every pediatric specialty, according to *U.S. News & World Report*.

Dr. Lawrence Stanberry succeeded Dr. Driscoll as department chair in 2008; the decade-long Stanberry legacy includes the era of molecular genetics, precision medicine, formation of the Columbia Children's Board, creation of the complex patient care program, faculty development and diversity initiatives, expansion of global health, and food insecurity programs.

One

THE HOLT YEARS

Born in 1855 in Upstate New York, Luther Emmett Holt graduated from College of Physicians and Surgeons (P&S), Columbia University, in 1878. After a surgical internship at Bellevue Hospital, he devoted his career to pediatrics. He became an editor of *Archives of Pediatrics*, the first journal devoted to children's diseases, and one of 43 charter members of the American Pediatric Society in 1887. Holt became the physician in chief of the Babies Hospital in 1888, upon the resignation of Sarah McNutt, and remained its leader until 1922. Under Holt's guidance, the Babies Hospital became the most celebrated pediatric hospital in the United States, and Holt became the foremost pediatrician in the country.

He authored a *Catechism for Nurses*, and in 1894, this was expanded and published as *The Care and Feeding of Children*. This text went through 75 printings, expanded to 200 pages, and was translated into scores of languages including Spanish, French, Russian, and Chinese.

In 1897, he completed a textbook of pediatrics, *Diseases of Infancy and Childhood*, recognized as the standard textbook of pediatrics and reprinted for 20 editions; in the same year, he was appointed president of the American Pediatric Society.

In 1902, the hospital moved to the corner of Fifty-Fifth Street and Lexington Avenue, where a modern seven-story building including outpatient facilities, laboratories, and 70 beds doubled the size of the original facility.

Holt was a favored lecturer and teacher at the College of Physicians and Surgeons of Columbia University; he became a professor of pediatrics at the medical school in 1901. Holt's teaching of medical students took the form of formal lectures held in the amphitheater of the medical school, formal clinics in the Vanderbilt Clinic, and informal clinic sessions at the Babies Hospital.

Holt's philosophy on child-rearing, a doctrine of conformity, dominated pediatric thinking and practice until the middle of the 20th century. The central concept is rigid and formulaic: fixed feeding hours, fixed sleeping habits, fixed dietary habits, strict reliance on maternal breast-feeding, and that each infant should be trained to conform to it.

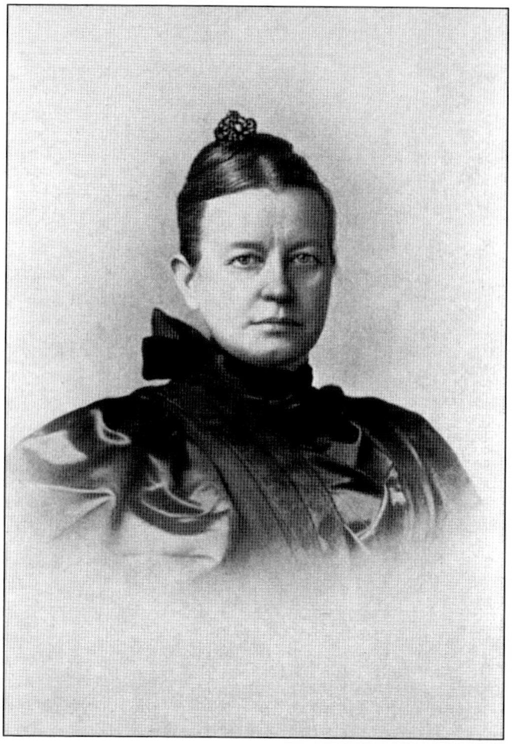

Sarah McNutt and her twin sister, Julia, were pioneering American female physicians and were among the five women who founded Babies Hospital in 1887 to provide medical and surgical aid and nursing for sick babies. Sarah (left) was born in Upstate New York in 1839 and received her medical degree from the Women's Medical College of the New York Infirmary in 1877. With Abraham Jacobi, she helped found the New York Post-Graduate Medical School, and she was the first woman elected to the American Neurological Association. McNutt died in Connecticut in 1930; about 85 years later, her medical school diploma was found hidden in the wall of a house there. The current owners generously donated it to Columbia University in recognition of McNutt's role as a founder of Babies Hospital. (Left, National Library of Medicine; below, Charles Manley.)

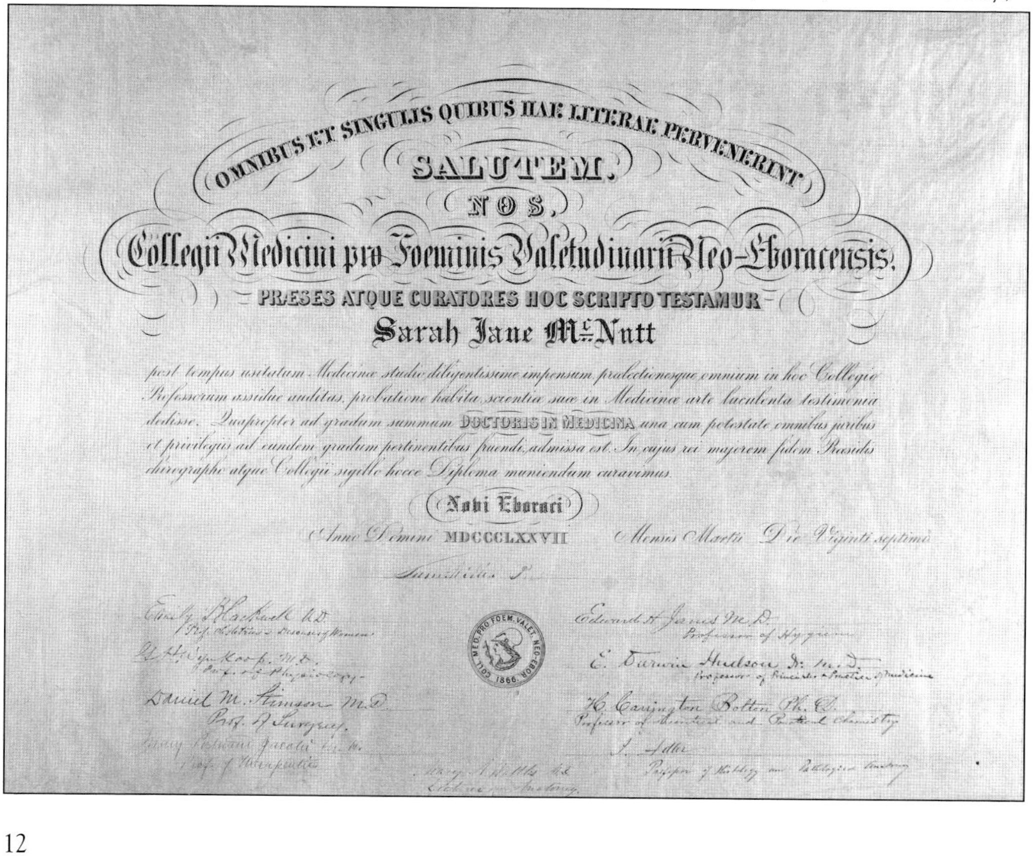

OMNIBUS ET SINGULIS QUIBUS HAE LITTERAE PERVENERINT
SALUTEM.
NOS,
Collegii Medicini pro Foeminis Valetudinarii Neo-Eboracensis,
PRESES ATQUE CURATORES HOC SCRIPTO TESTAMUR
Sarah Jane McNutt
post tempus usitatum Medicinae studio diligentissime impensum, praelectionesque omnium in hoc Collegio Professorum assidue auditas, probatione habita, scientiae suae in Medicinae arte luculenta testimonia dedisse. Quapropter ad gradum summum DOCTORIS IN MEDICINA una cum potestate omnibus juribus et privilegiis ad eundem gradum pertinentibus fruendi, admissa est. In cujus rei majorem fidem Praesidis chirographo atque Collegii sigillo hocce Diploma muniendum curavimus.
Novi Eboraci
Anno Domini MDCCCLXXVII Mensis Martii Die Viginti septimo

A year after its founding in 1887, Babies Hospital purchased its first permanent home, a brownstone at the northeast corner of East Fifty-Fifth Street and Lexington Avenue. In 1894, it acquired the adjoining residence. Even then, the buildings were recognized as being too small, and annual reports at the time complained about the lack of a proper operating rooms and other inadequacies. The photograph below shows the Nicholas Gwynn Ward about 1895. Clearly a converted brownstone room, the long, narrow space would have lacked much light and appears to have fewer than 10 beds. However, these deficiencies did not prevent the hospital from treating 425 patients that year, and with all these shortcomings, the buildings remained the hospital's home until a new structure was erected on the site in 1902.

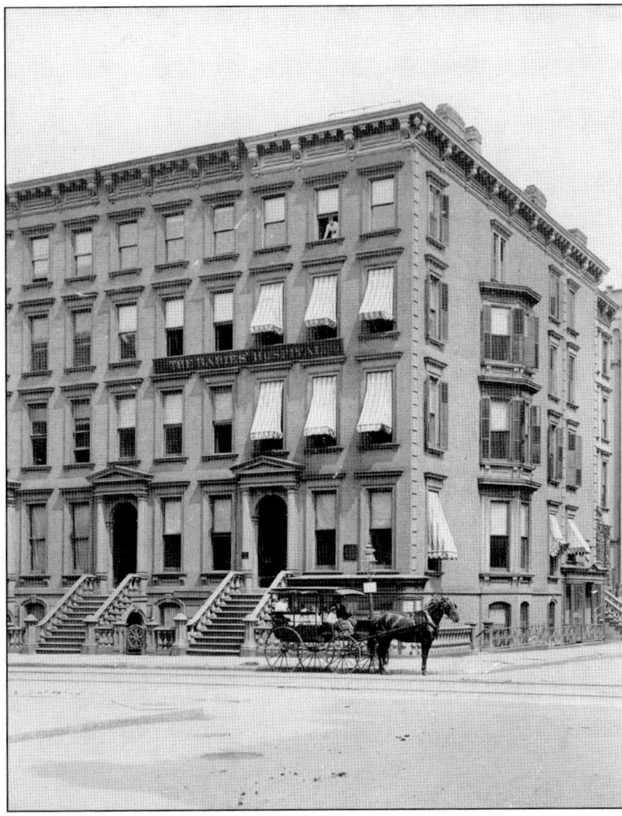

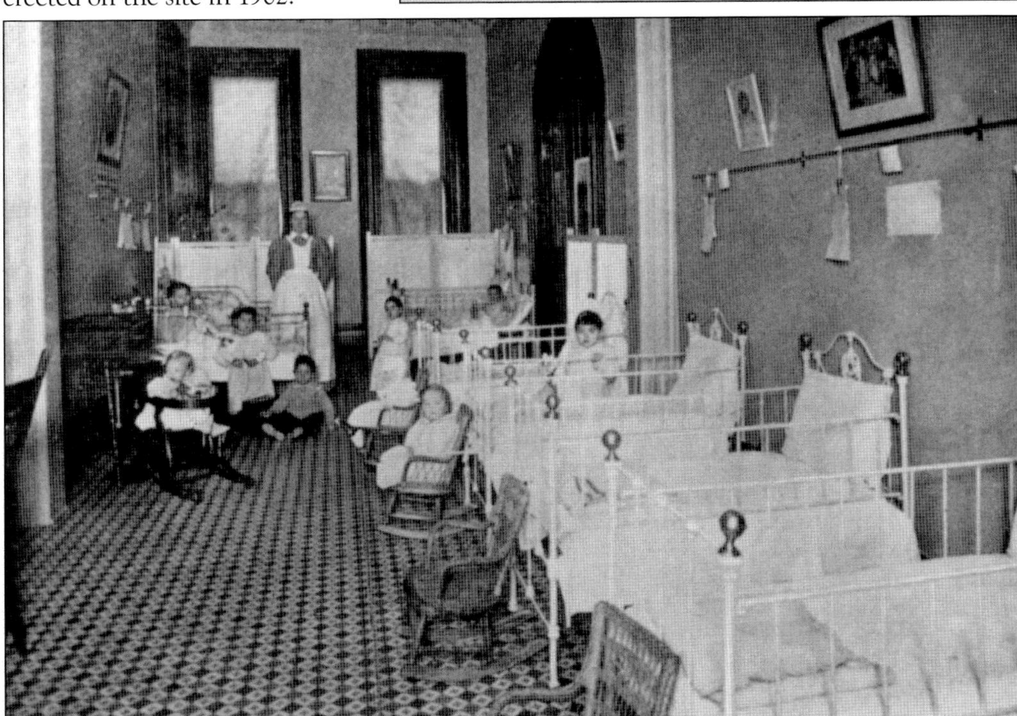

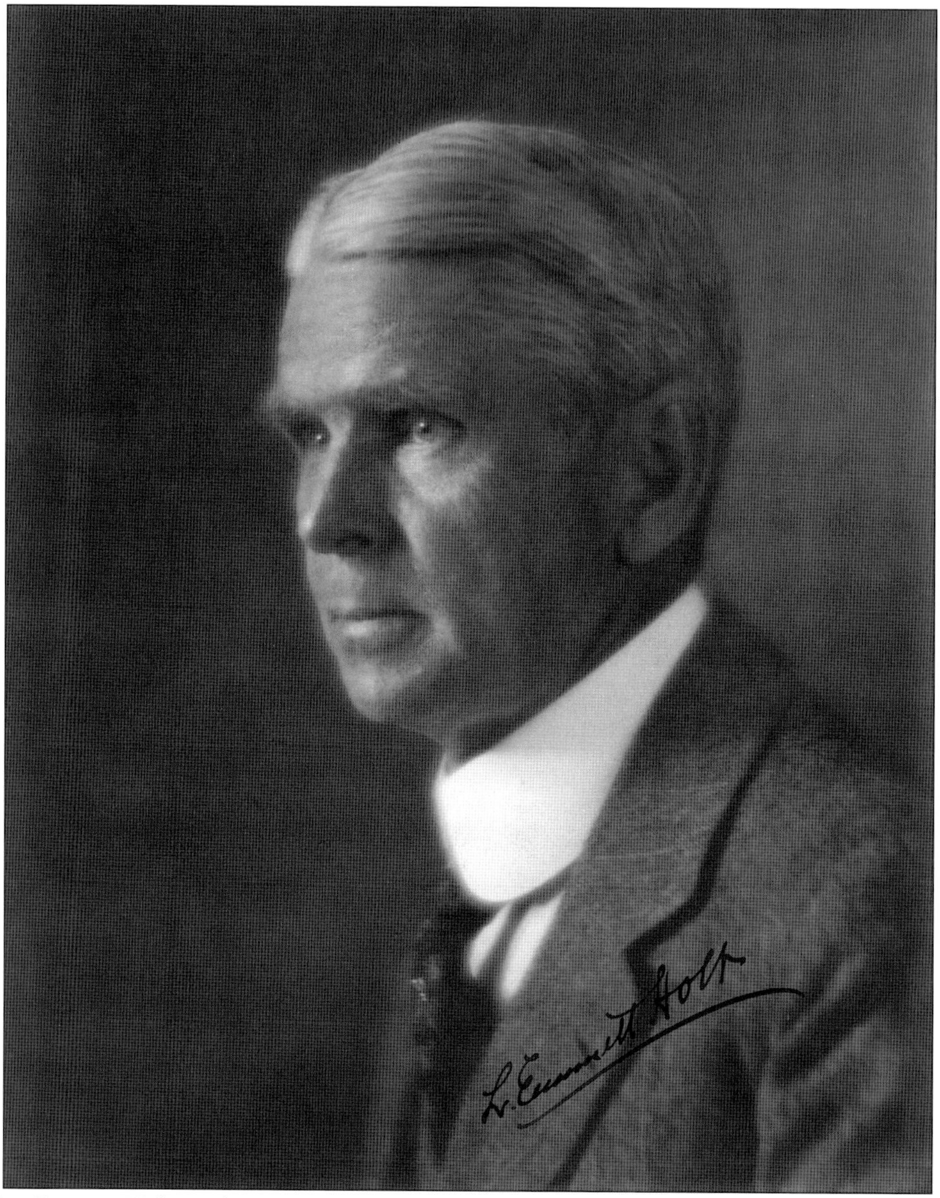

Luther Emmett Holt was born in Upstate New York and received his undergraduate education at the University of Rochester. He graduated from Columbia's College of Physicians and Surgeons in 1880 and then did an internship at Bellevue Hospital. At first interested in orthopedic surgery, Holt's focus soon shifted to pediatrics. He became director of Babies Hospital in 1888 after Sarah McNutt stepped down and served until 1922. In the meantime, he became one of the most influential American pediatricians of his day. His *Catechism for Nurses*, a manual he wrote for the instruction of the Babies Hospital staff, was published as *The Care and Feeding of Children* in 1894. It became a worldwide best seller, going through 75 editions and numerous translations. His textbook *Diseases of Infancy and Childhood* (1896) became the definitive work on the subject in English and went through 20 editions. He was a mentor to many of the notable pediatricians of the next generation. Holt died in 1924 in Beijing while a visiting lecturer at the Rockefeller Foundation's new medical college.

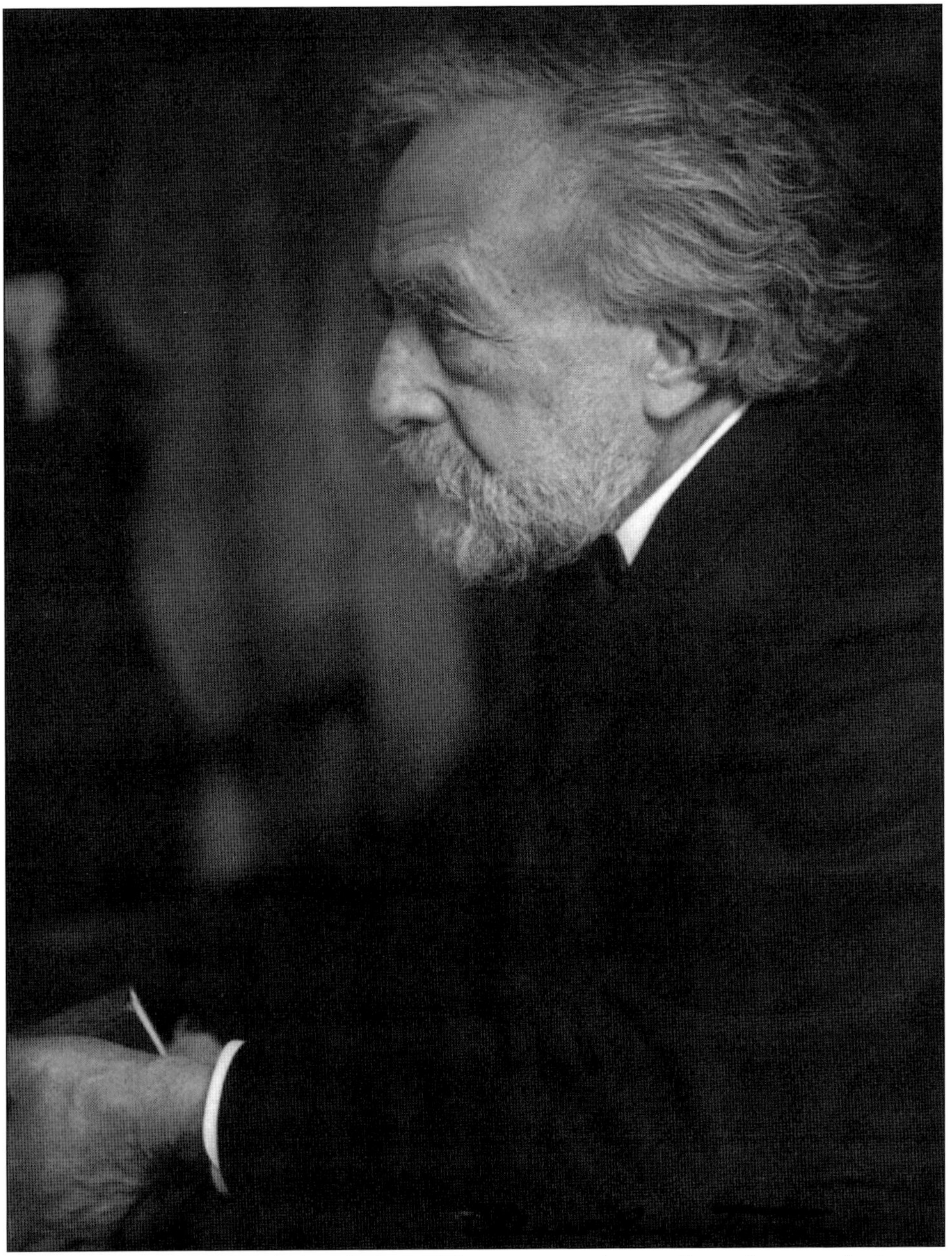

Abraham Jacobi, considered the "father of American pediatrics," was born and educated in Germany. After involvement in the failed revolution of 1848, he was imprisoned for treason. Upon his release in 1853, he immigrated to Britain, where he became friends with Karl Marx and Friedrich Engels. The next year, he moved to New York, where he became one of the city's best-known physicians and a leading expert on the diseases of children. He taught at numerous medical schools, including New York Medical College, New York University, and Columbia's College of Physicians and Surgeons, where he was a professor of pediatrics for over 30 years. Jacobi Medical Center in the Bronx is named in his honor. Although not involved in the founding of Babies Hospital, Jacobi early joined its staff. He was both consulting physician and president of the medical board for over a quarter-century.

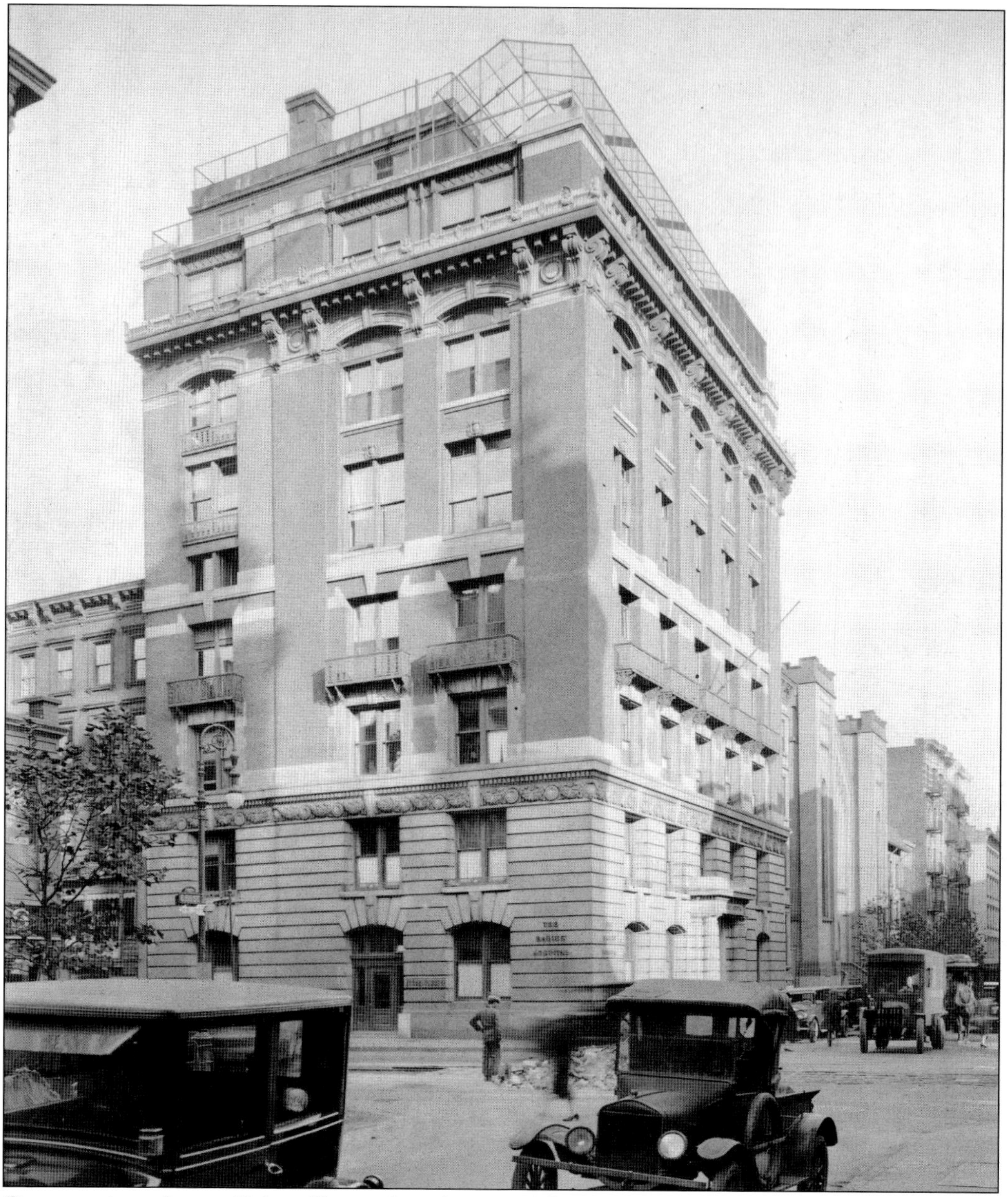

Construction of a new Babies Hospital on the site of the existing buildings began in August 1901. The work went swiftly, and the structure was ready for occupancy in December 1902. Designed by the well-known architectural firm of York & Sawyer, the new hospital had seven and a half stories over a full basement and was constructed of limestone and brick. It included five spacious wards accommodating 55 beds, quarters for nurses and residents, a laboratory, a chapel, and a solarium. The cost came to a little over $48,000, equal to $1.5 million today. Among the donors to the building fund were many of the wealthiest families of Gilded Age New York. Mrs. Andrew Carnegie (Louise) gave $5,000, as did John D. Rockefeller Sr. and banker Felix Warburg. Mrs. Cornelius Vanderbilt (Alice) donated $1,000, while Macy's owner and *Titanic* victim Isidor Straus gave $500. Remarkably, considering how quickly New York City streetscapes change, this building still exists at the corner of Lexington Avenue and East Fifty-Fifth Street.

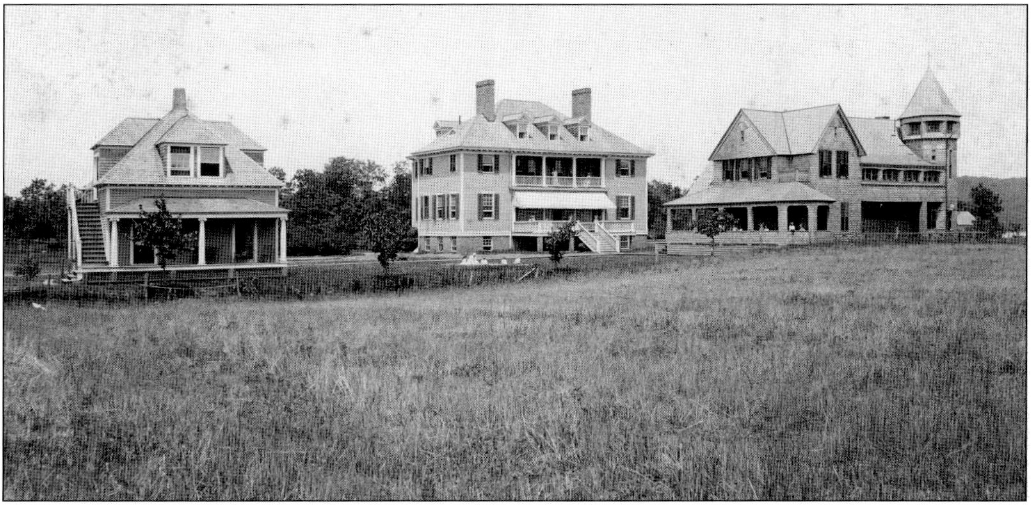

From 1888 through 1931, Babies Hospital operated a "Summer Hospital" on the New Jersey shore at Rumson, where patients needing the cooling breezes and fresh air of the seaside could convalesce. Many were suffering from the then common gastrointestinal disease known as "summer diarrhea." By 1895, a three-building campus had been erected. Seen above, from left to right, are the Reception Cottage, where children with infectious diseases were isolated; the hospital, which included three wards and accommodations for staff; and the Hamersley Cottage for older children. Both the hospital building and the Hamersley Cottage were given in memory of the deceased children of the donors, showing that even the wealthy were not spared the high child mortality of the period. In the photograph below, a nurse supervises the Robbins Ward in the hospital.

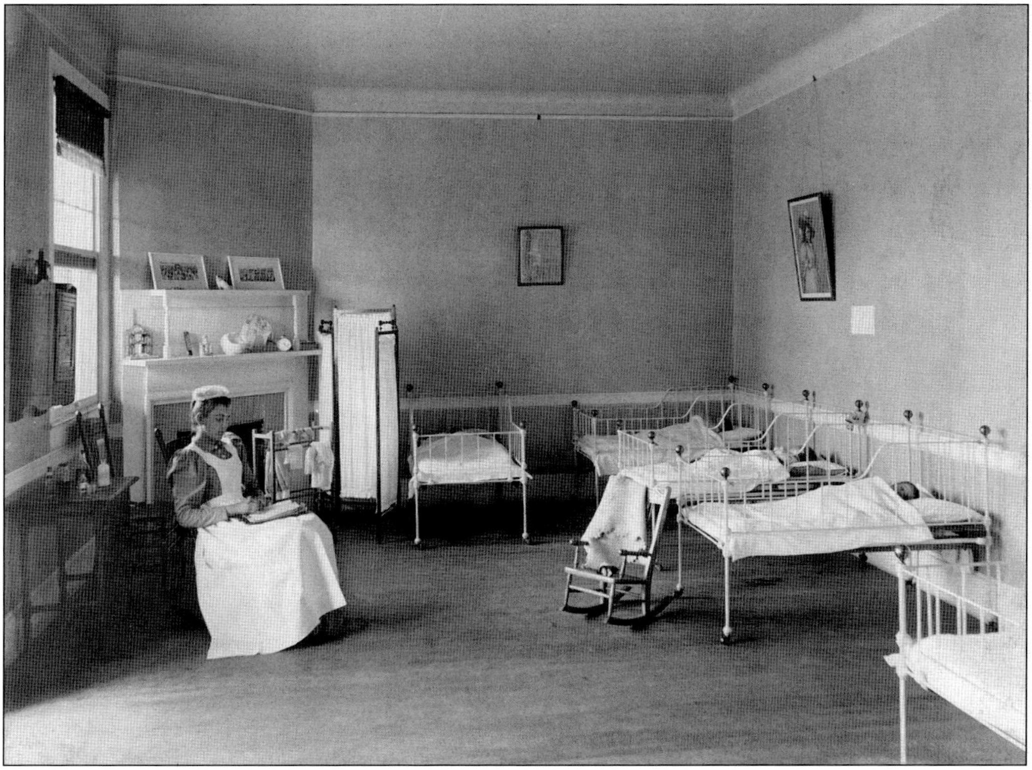

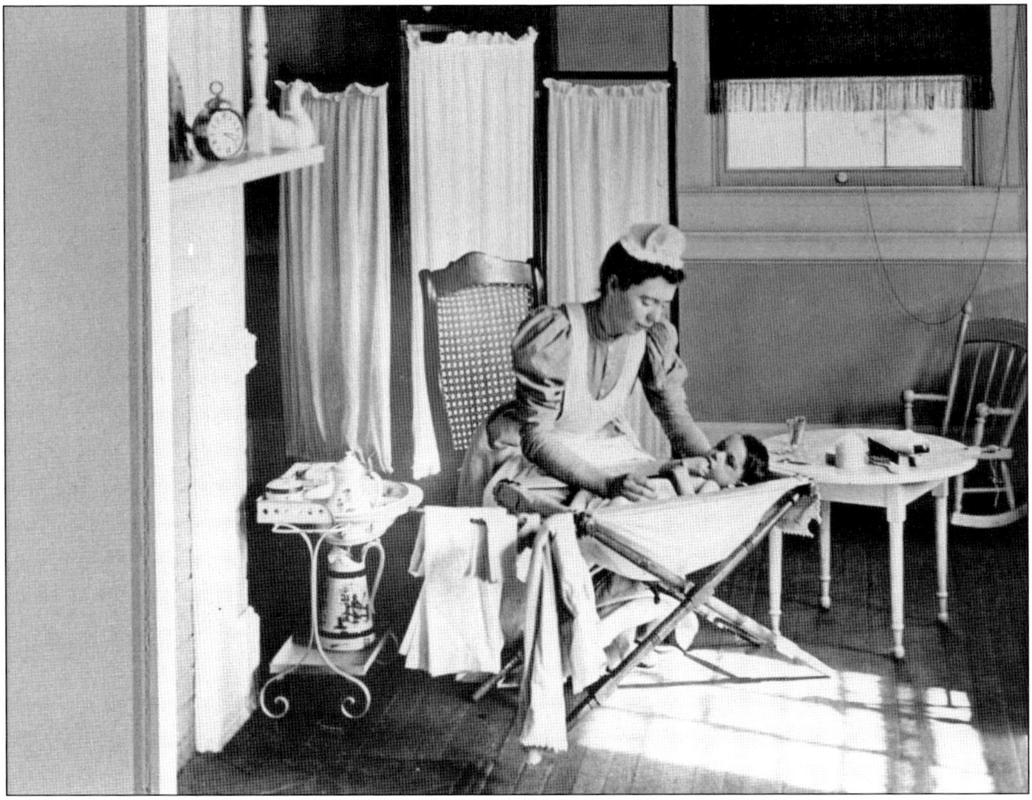

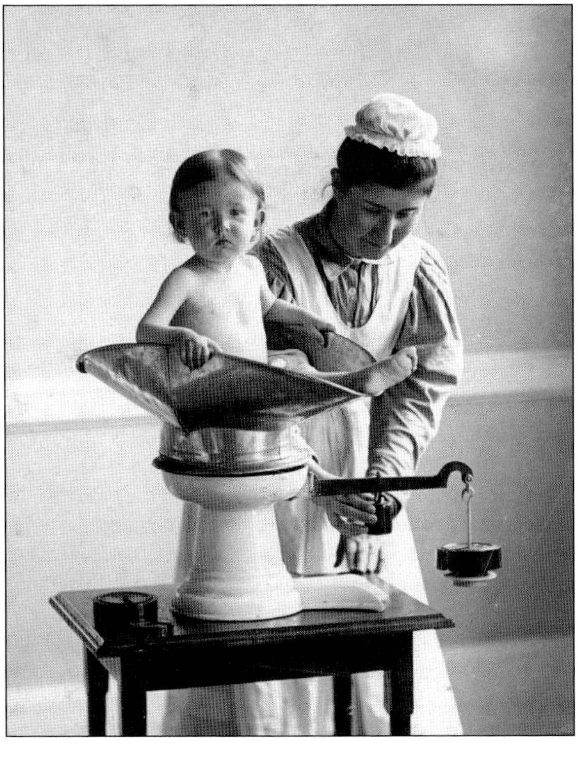

From 1889 to 1942, Babies Hospital ran a Training School for Nursery Maids to train young women "who desire to go out to service to care for infants and young children" (Annual Report, 1891). Students learned on the job, providing much of the nursing care at Babies Hospital, as seen in these images from early annual reports. Instruction included infant feeding, bathing, hygiene of the skin, care of the mouth, eyes, and ears, nursery hygiene, simple emergency treatments, and elements of kindergarten work. Originally four months long, the course expanded over the decades and, by 1934, took a full year. After 1898, students received $5 a month for the first five months and $12 for the last month and were guaranteed $20 a month for their first six months of employment.

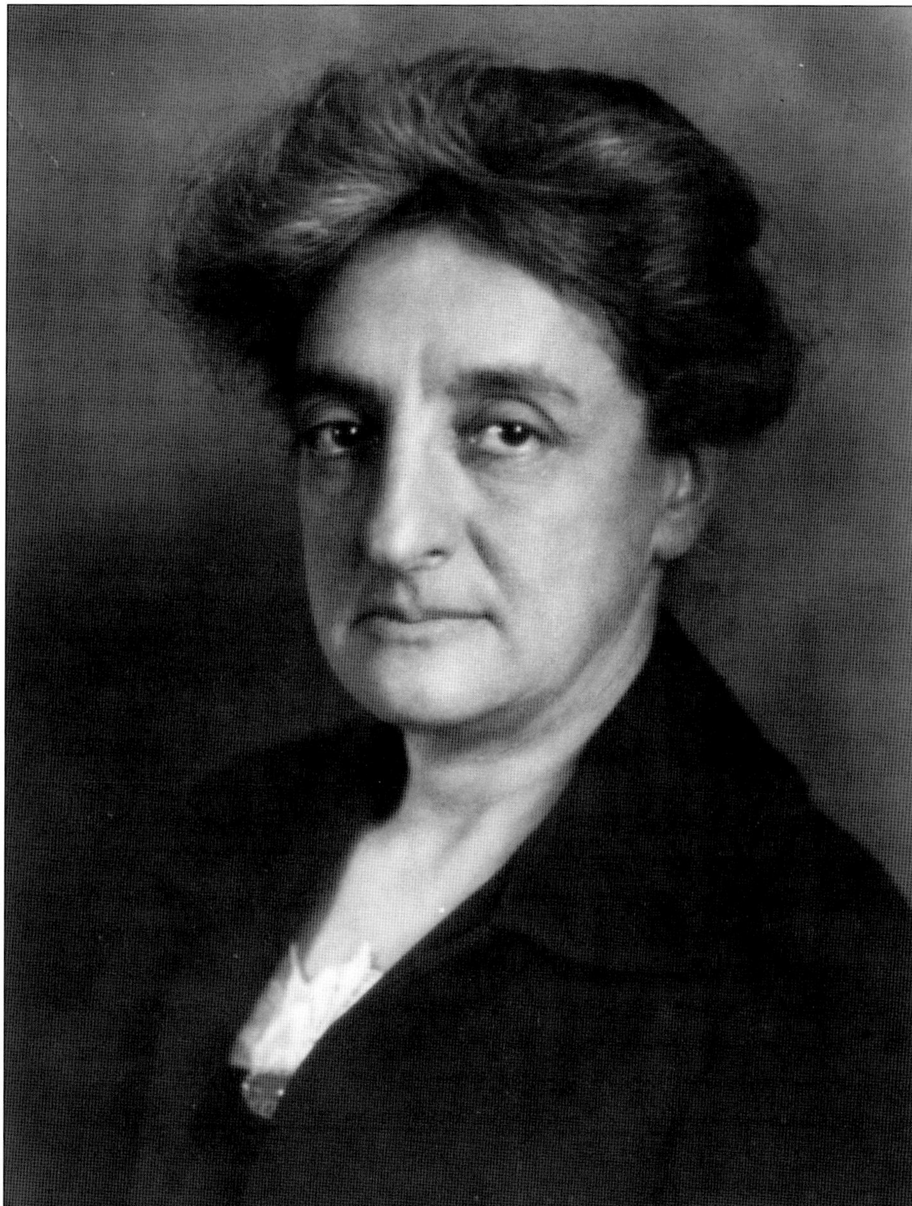

Dr. Martha Wollstein, the first pediatric pathologist in the United States, spent her entire 45-year career, from 1891 to 1935, at Babies Hospital. She received her medical degree from the Woman's Medical College of the New York Infirmary, where she studied with the famed Mary Putnam Jacobi. In 1889, Dr. Wollstein was appointed as the very first resident at Babies Hospital, and in 1901, she was named the hospital's first pathologist. Wollstein was certainly the first fully specialized pediatric perinatal pathologist practicing at a children's hospital in North America. She practiced the full scope of hospital pathology, including anatomical pathology, microbiology, and hematology. Dr. Wollstein became an expert in congenital heart disease and focused on the anatomy of disease in early life with an emphasis on pediatric infectious diseases. Among her important findings was her research indicating that the underlying cause of mumps is a virus. In 1930, she was the first woman elected as a member of the American Pediatric Society.

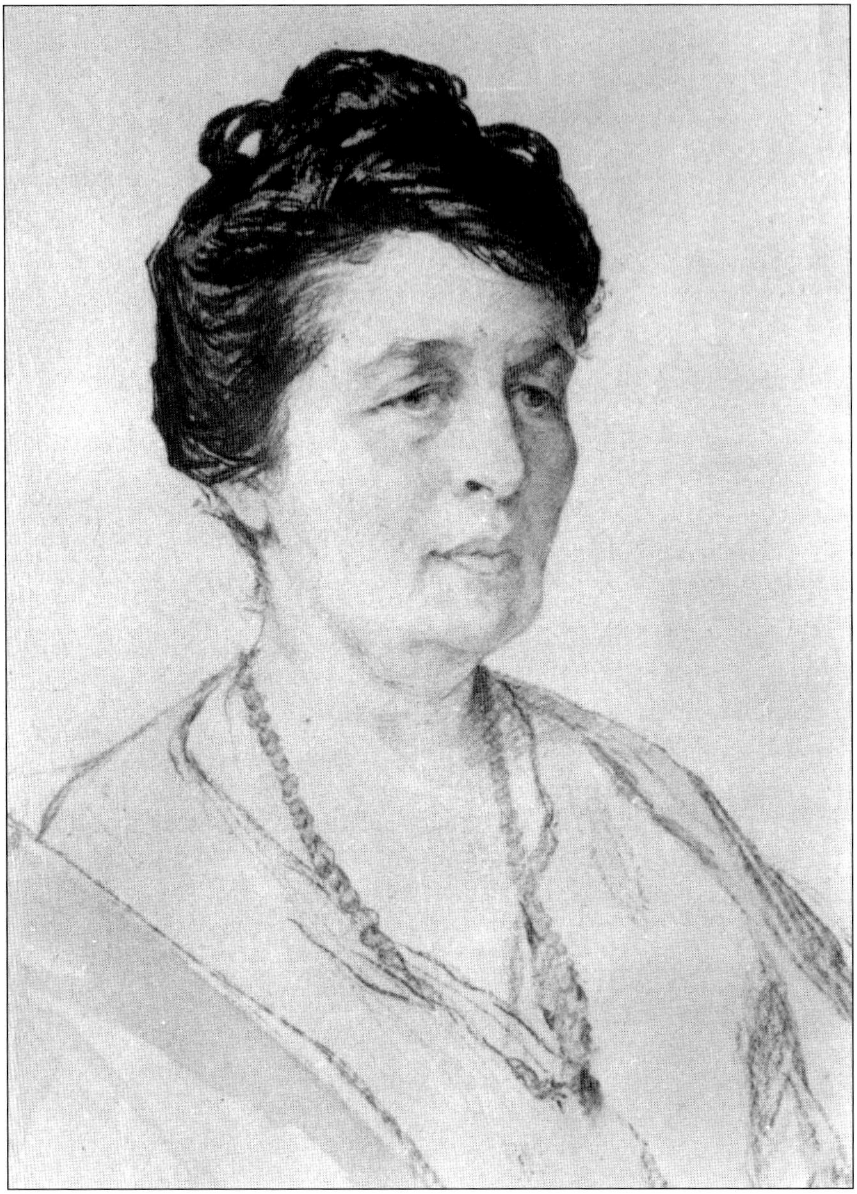

Dorothy Reed, MD, completed undergraduate studies at Smith College and graduated fourth in her class from the Johns Hopkins University School of Medicine in 1900. The famed Hopkins physician Dr. William Osler told her "medicine is not a place for women" and that a medical education was "wasted on women." Not discouraged, Reed accepted an internship in pediatrics at the Babies Hospital in New York City; arguably, she was the first resident physician to have worked under the direction of L. Emmett Holt. Dr. Reed developed particular expertise in pathology. In 1901, at only 28 years of age, she made her most recognized contribution to medical science, the discovery of the Reed-Sternberg cell, which she identified as a diagnostic marker for Hodgkin's lymphoma. This cell would initially be named the Dorothy Reed Cell before later being called the Reed-Sternberg cell. Dorothy Reed Mendenhall, as she was known after her 1906 marriage to Charles E. Mendenhall, a fellow Hopkins medical student, spent her professional career at the University of Wisconsin, where she became an expert in maternal and infant health.

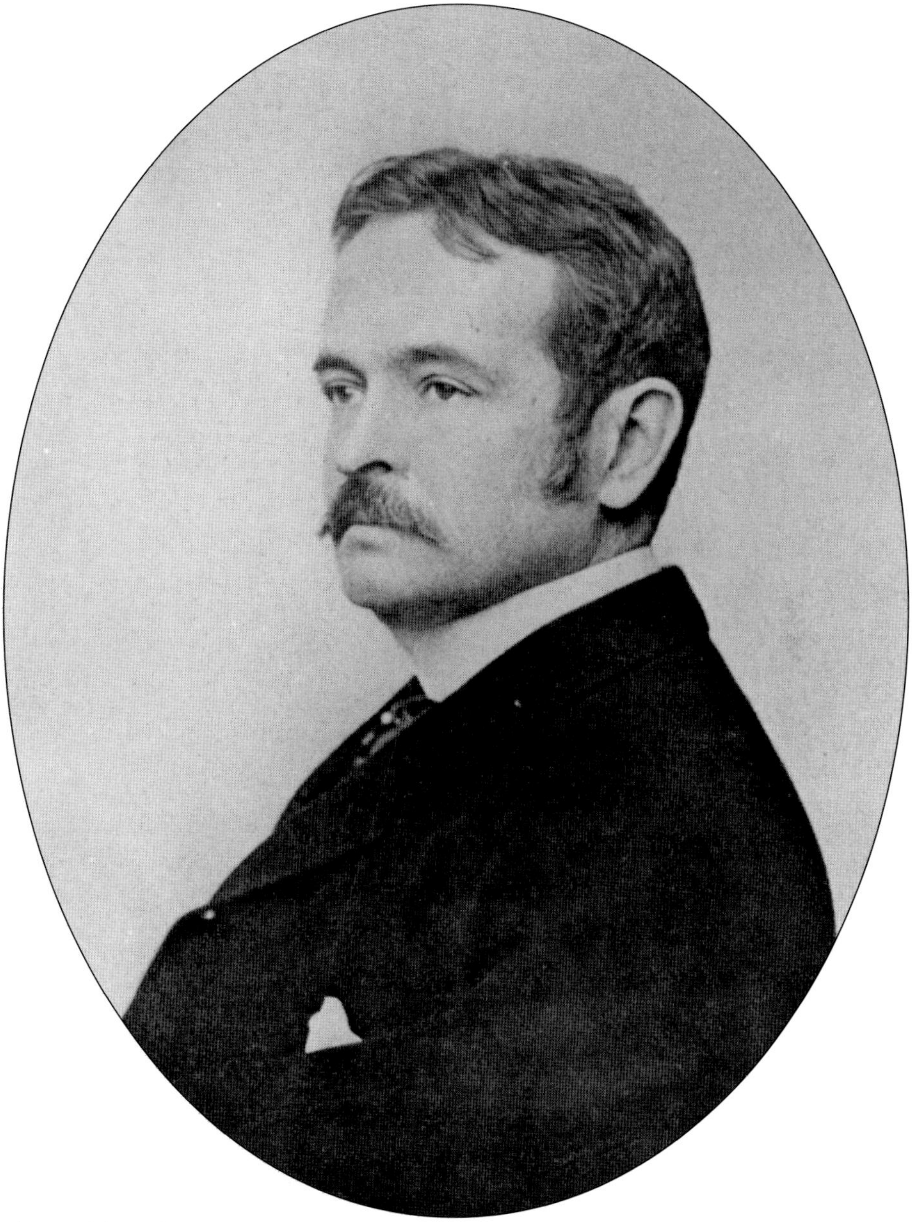

Dr. Robert Abbe, who received his medical degree from the Columbia University College of Physicians and Surgeons in 1874, was both a general and plastic surgeon, an attending surgeon at Babies Hospital, and a pioneering radiologist. In 1892, he performed perhaps the first recorded nephrectomy, removing a two-pound tumor from the kidney of an eight-month-old child. The following year, he removed a 7.5-pound kidney tumor from a 14-month-old. Abbe befriended Marie Curie, the codiscoverer of radium, and explored the medical uses of radiation and x-rays. In 1904, he introduced in the United States the use of radiation to treat cancer, and he is credited as the founder of radiation oncology in America. He was a vigorous opponent of tobacco, which he considered a cause of cancer, and reported more than 100 cases of smoker's cancer. Besides his work at Babies Hospital, Abbe taught surgery at Columbia, the Women's Medical College, and the New York Post-Graduate Medical School.

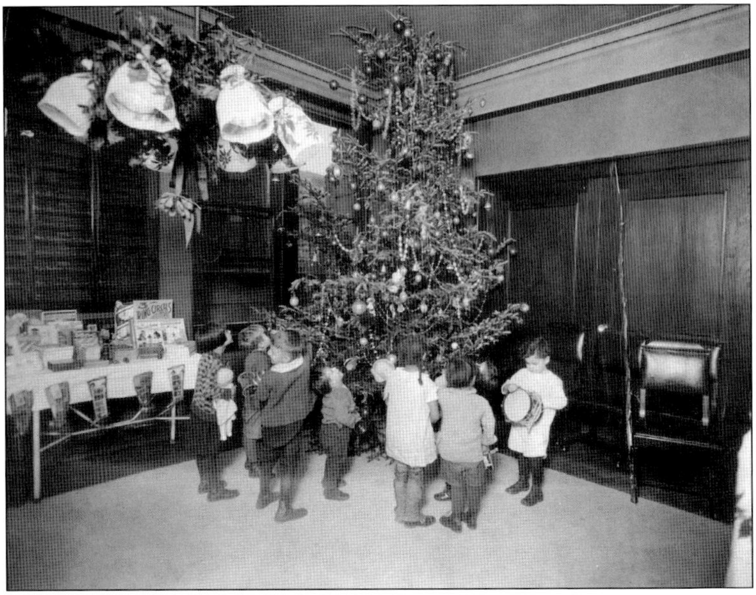

The hospital has always tried to make Christmas a joyous occasion for its patients who find themselves separated from family during this festive time of year. Just because they are hospitalized does not mean Santa has forgotten them. Here, patients gaze in wonder at the towering Christmas tree or grasp their new presents during the 1926 party at the Fifty-Fifth Street hospital.

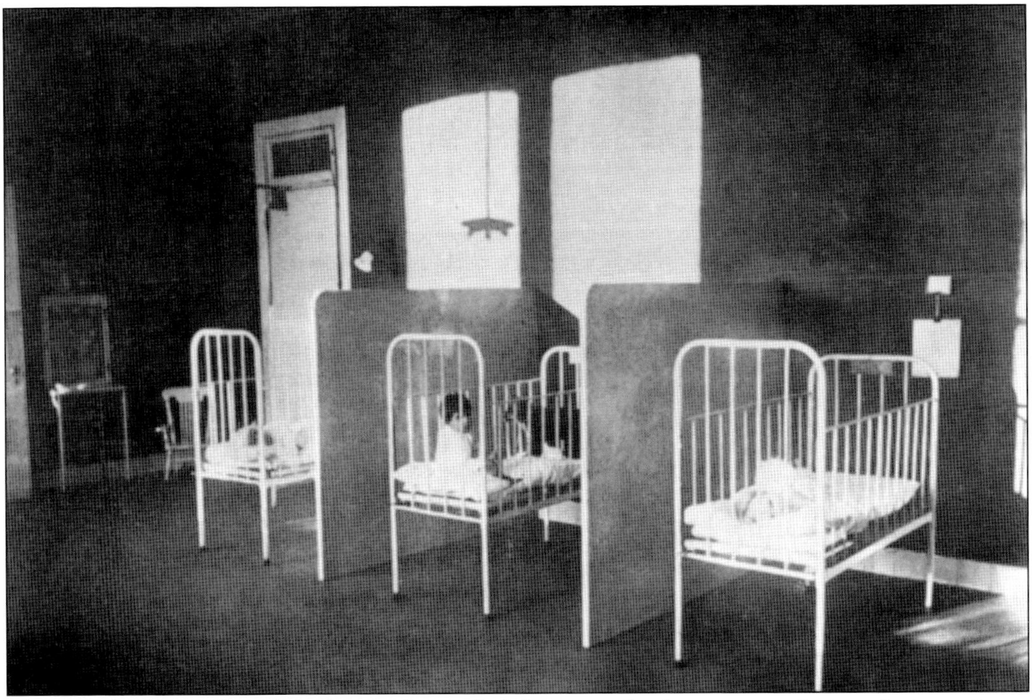

The 1902 building allowed the hospital to include better and safer accommodations for its patients. Shown here is the isolation ward, which the hospital's 1910 annual report described as a "ward which is designed to prevent bed-to-bed infection, accomplished by the erection of marble slabs, forming alcoves. Excellent results have come from this experiment."

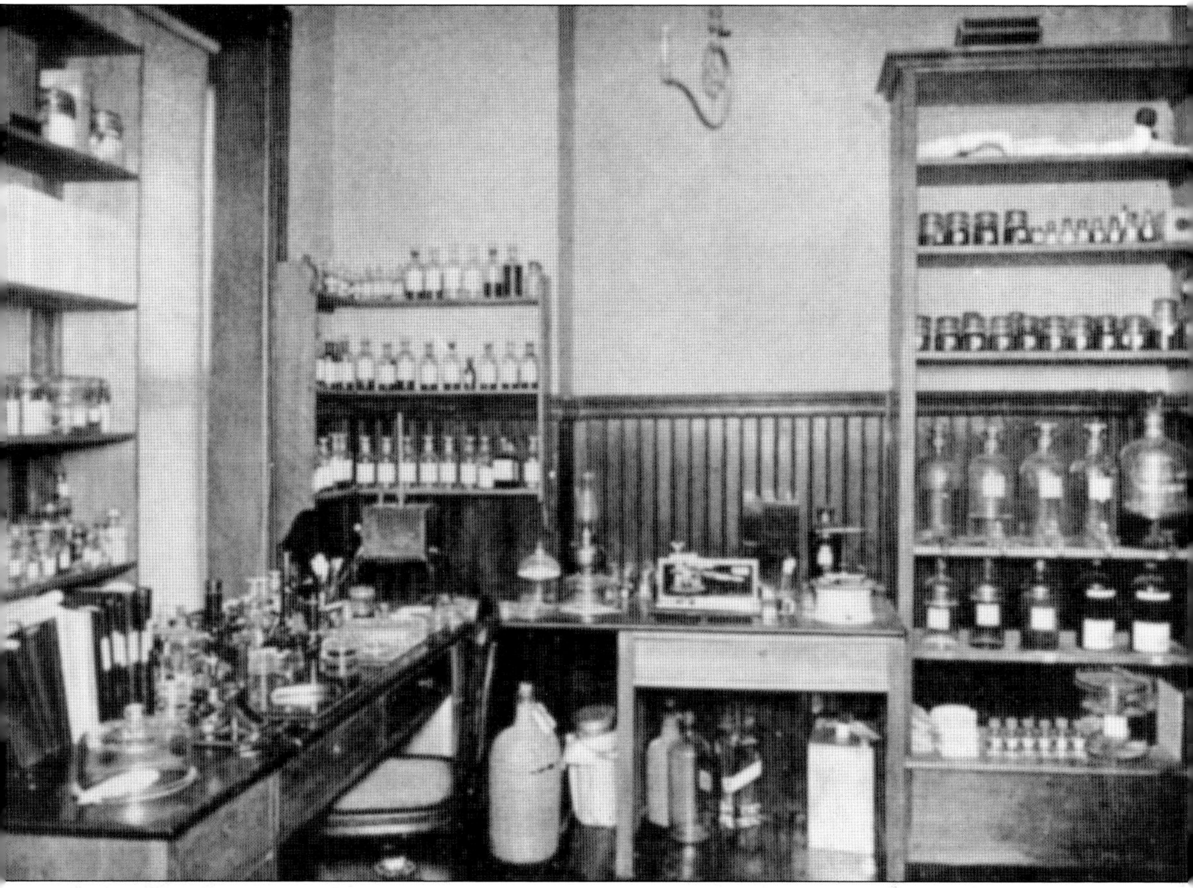

Babies Hospital's first laboratory was a gift from Dr. Christian A. Herter, one of its consulting physicians. In 1896, he donated funds to establish the facility and pay the salary of an assistant. The hospital's 1897 annual report noted that the laboratory "has made possible a more thorough and exhaustive study of cases in the Hospital, and has furnished an opportunity for the prosecution of regular scientific work in the investigation of many phases of infancy and childhood which can be studied nowhere else than in a Hospital like this. . . . Here also our milk supply is watched and regular examinations made to insure its richness, purity and cleanliness. In short, the laboratory has become almost the right arm of hospital service." The annual report went on to say that "much has already been published from the Hospital, both in clinical reports and the results of laboratory work, and much more will now be possible than ever before." Dr. Herter continued to support the laboratory out of his own pocket for many years.

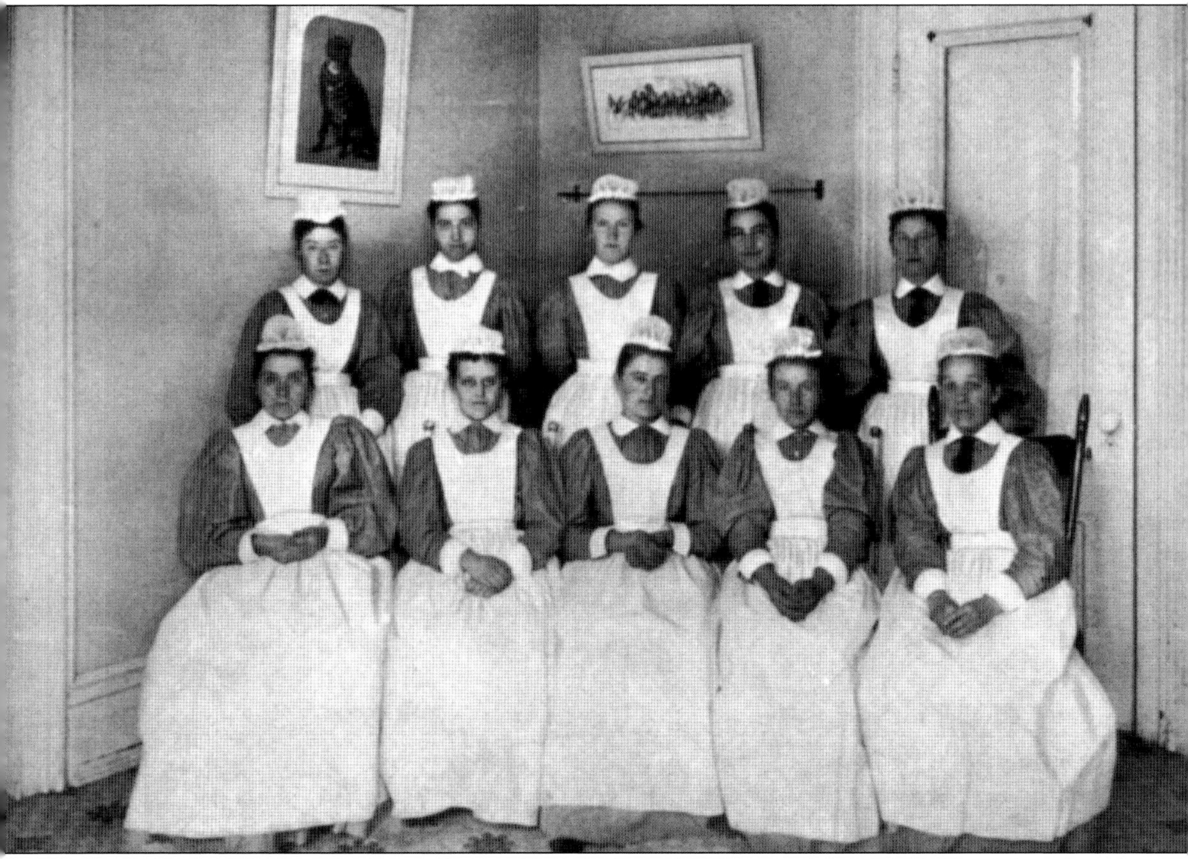

Members of the 1896–1897 "mid-year class" of the Babies Hospital Training School for Nursery Maids pose for their group portrait. That year's annual report noted "the good work still goes on, and if the demand for well-trained, efficient Nursery Maids is a criterion from which to judge the character of the work in hand, we certainly have reason to feel that our efforts are not in vain." The report went on to say, "this subject of preparing nurses for the care of children is becoming an important one and we feel more convinced each year that the old idea that any person could 'mind the baby,' is about exhausted, and certainly an injustice to the little ones sent to brighten our homes." By that year, the school had graduated 90 nurses and had a waiting list of 15 applicants. The annual report expressed concern at the school's lack of space, "but the fact that the results obtained have been appreciated by so many mothers and guardians of children has encouraged us."

Two

The Wilcox Years

Herbert Wilcox succeeded L. Emmett Holt as the director of the Babies Hospital and pediatrician-in-chief in 1922. He was born in Brooklyn, completed his undergraduate degree at Yale University, and gained his medical degree from the College of Physicians and Surgeons of Columbia University in 1902.

In 1929, Wilcox was responsible for the relocation of the Babies Hospital from Lexington Avenue and Fifty-Fifth Street to a new building on the campus of the Columbia-Presbyterian Medical Center on Broadway and West 168th Street. The new hospital site had previously been called the American League Park, also known as Hilltop Park, home to the New York Highlanders baseball team from 1903 until 1912. Diana Rice of the *New York Times* referred to the facility as "the last word in hospital design and equipment." The 12-story building was designed to accommodate a variety of programs related to children's health care, including private and shared patient rooms, a nurse training center, a nurse dormitory, classrooms for medical students, playrooms, solariums, a roof garden, and paneled administrative facilities.

The hospital was socially progressive. Children of all racial and socioeconomic backgrounds were cared for in the same place. This principle and dedication to diversity date back to 1890, as the original Babies Hospital mission statement and rules indicated that no patient was too ill or too poor to receive care.

Wilcox was responsible for a rapid expansion of established departments as well as instituting new initiatives. The new hospital had 190 beds and accepted children up to and including 12 years of age. Specialists on staff now included surgery, bacteriology, chemistry, dermatology, neurology, radiology, ophthalmology, orthopedics, otolaryngology, pathology, urology, and anesthesiology. The pathology department expanded to include laboratories for hematology, microbiology, and chemistry. Clinics were established in the Vanderbilt Clinic for children with asthma and eczema. In conjunction with the departments of medicine and neurology, a new clinic for convulsive disorders was started. A surgery clinic, eye clinic, skin clinic, vaccination clinic, and programs for posture, massage, and heliotherapy were also provided.

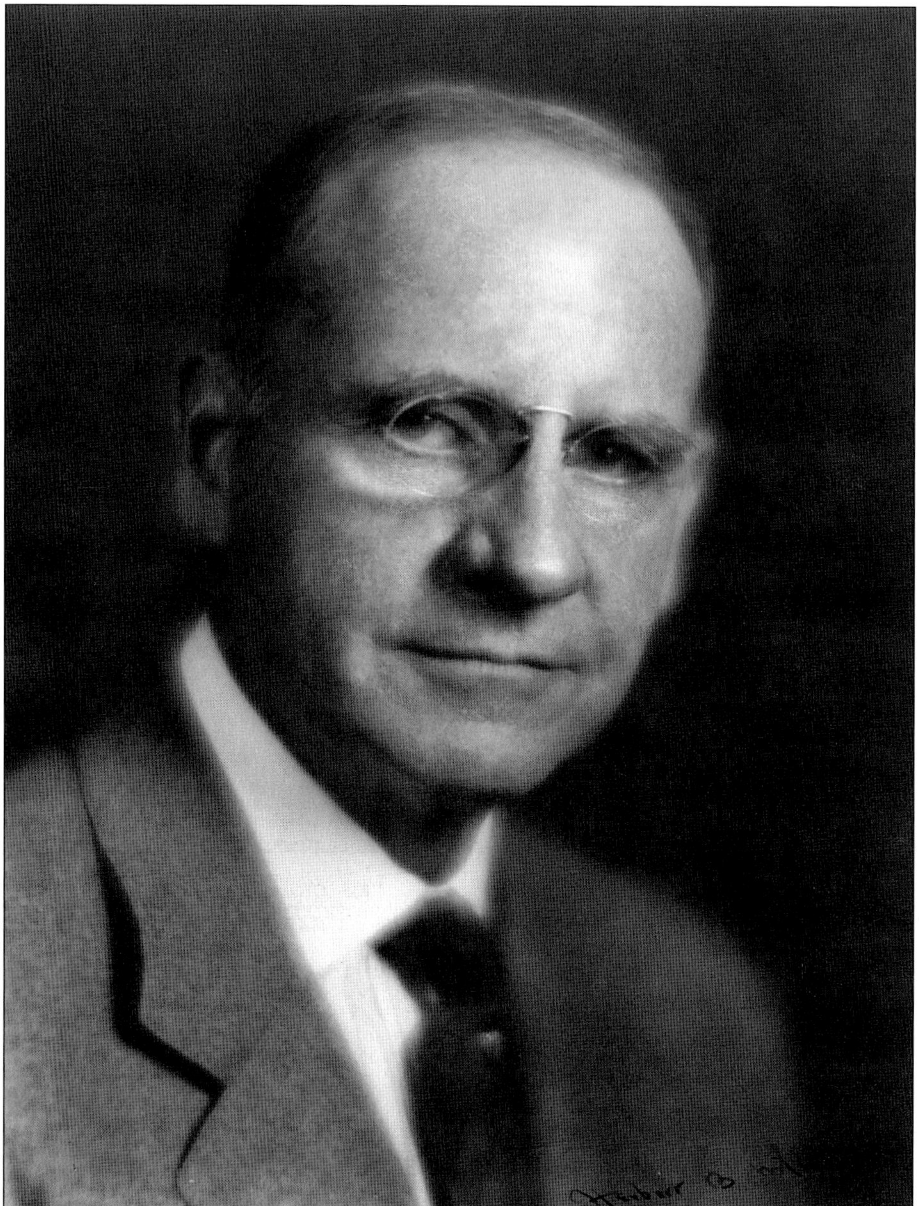

Herbert Budington Wilcox graduated from the College of Physicians and Surgeons of Columbia University in 1902. Although initially trained as an internist, Wilcox practiced pediatrics for his entire career. He served as the director of the Children's Medical Division at Bellevue Hospital for several years and then, in 1922, succeeded L. Emmett Holt as both the physician-in-chief at Babies Hospital and the Carpentier Professor of Pediatrics at Columbia's College of Physicians and Surgeons. Wilcox was keenly aware of the benefit to the Babies Hospital of becoming part of the Columbia-Presbyterian Medical Center and worked tirelessly to achieve this goal. During his tenure, the construction of the Babies Hospital on the Washington Heights campus of the medical center was completed in 1929. Wilcox served as president of the American Pediatric Society, and after his retirement from Babies Hospital, he became director of the New York Academy of Medicine.

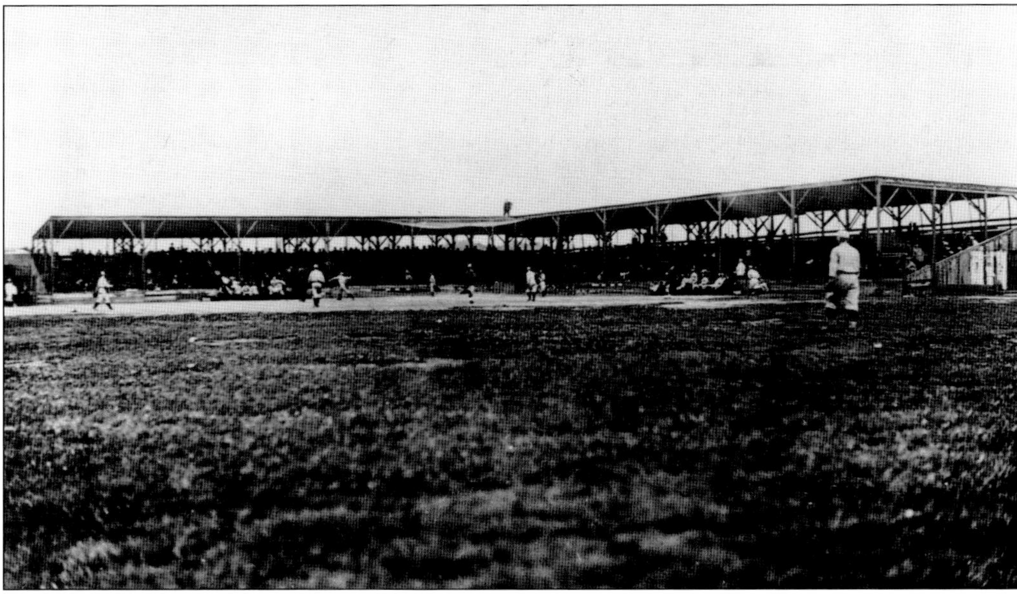

Hilltop Park was the first home of the New York Highlanders, now better known as the New York Yankees. The team occupied the site of the current Columbia University Irving Medical Center from 1903 to 1912. After the stadium's demolition in 1914, the site was purchased by philanthropist and Presbyterian Hospital trustee Edward Harkness to be the location of the world's first academic medical center, Columbia-Presbyterian, which opened in 1928. On September 30, 1993, a plaque, seen below, was placed on the hospital grounds to mark the former location of home plate in Hilltop Park. Donated to the hospital by the New York Yankees, the plaque commemorates the exact location where home plate rested in their first home. (Below, photograph by Joan Penn.)

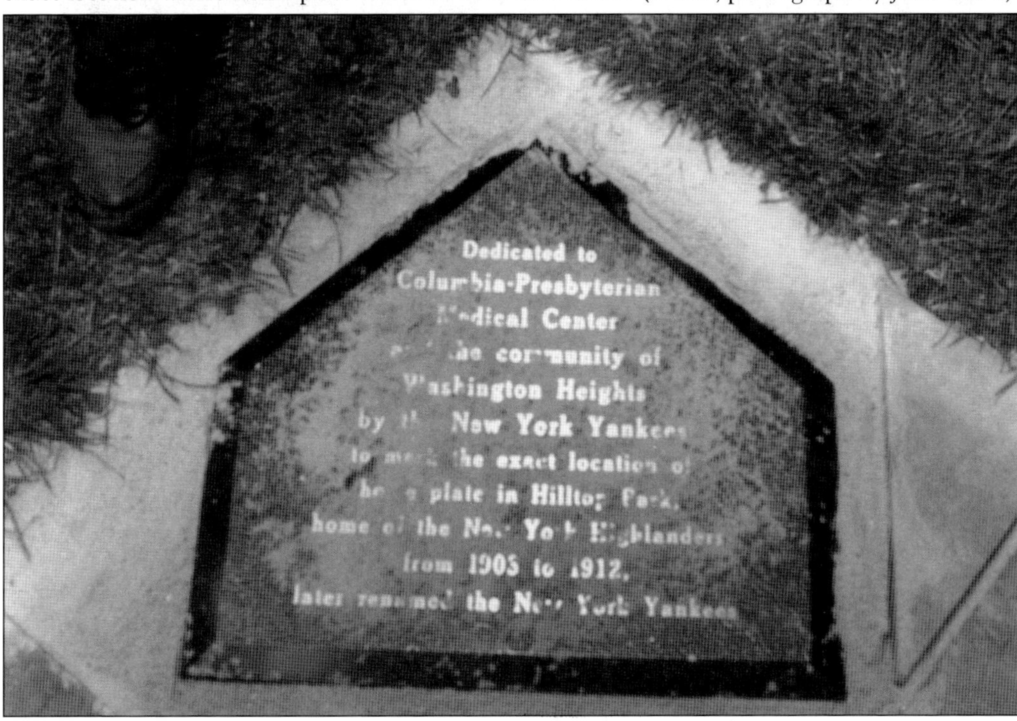

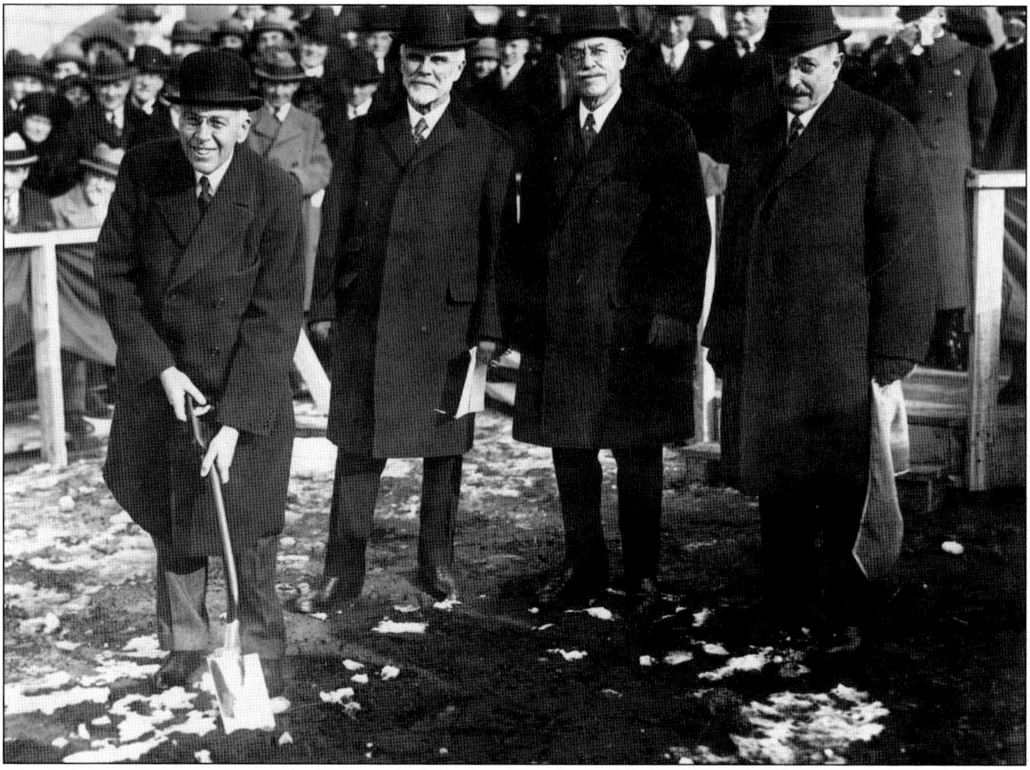

The Columbia University College of Physicians and Surgeons and Presbyterian Hospital allied in 1911 to form a medical center that would combine research, medical education, and patient care in one complex. However, due to fund-raising issues and World War I, it took 14 years before construction could begin. On January 31, 1925, the ground was broken for what would become the Columbia-Presbyterian Medical Center (now the Columbia University Irving Medical Center). Above, Edward S. Harkness, a Presbyterian board member and major donor, wields the first shovelful of earth. Once begun, construction was rapid. By December 29 of that year, much of the steelwork for the new complex was in place (below). Seeing that the medical center was now a viable project, Babies Hospital joined it as its pediatric component in 1925, though it retained its autonomy. (Both photographs by Underwood & Underwood.)

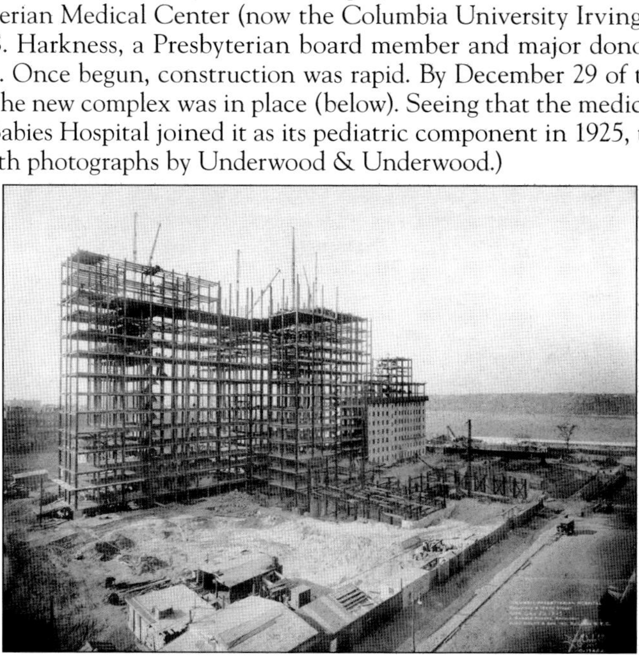

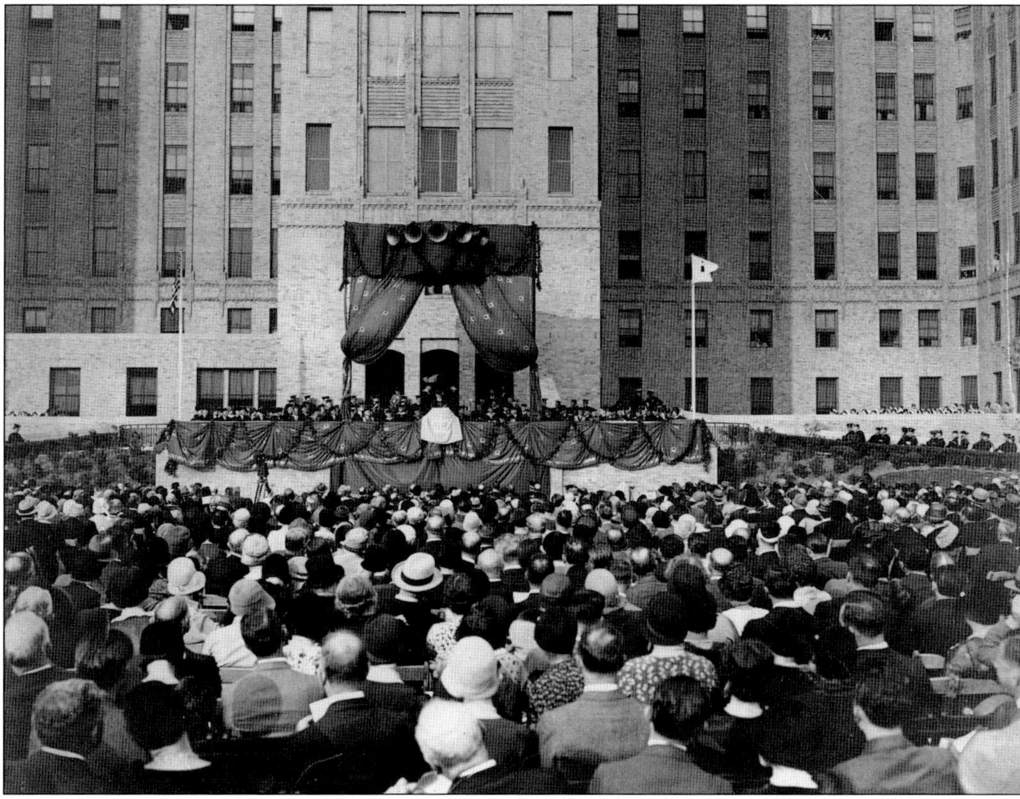

The formal dedication of the Columbia-Presbyterian Medical Center was held on October 12, 1928, amid pomp and ceremony. A crowd of over 3,000 assembled in the medical center garden in unusually warm weather to witness the proceedings (above). Columbia University president Nicholas Murray Butler conferred honorary degrees on the four men most responsible for seeing the project to fruition: philanthropist Edward S. Harkness, architect James Gamble Rogers, Presbyterian Hospital president Dean Sage, and contractor Otto Eidlitz. The audience then heard Samuel W. Lambert, dean emeritus of Columbia's medical school (below), deliver an address in which he declared "these buildings of the Medical Centre present the latest fulfillment which has built to carry out the complex requirements of an art and a science." (Both photographs by Underwood & Underwood.)

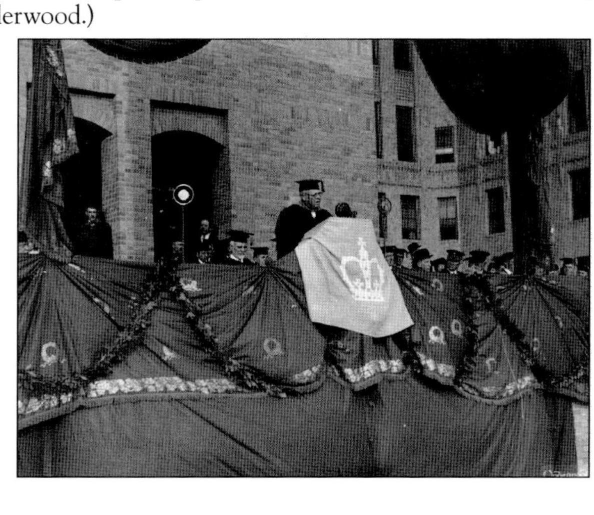

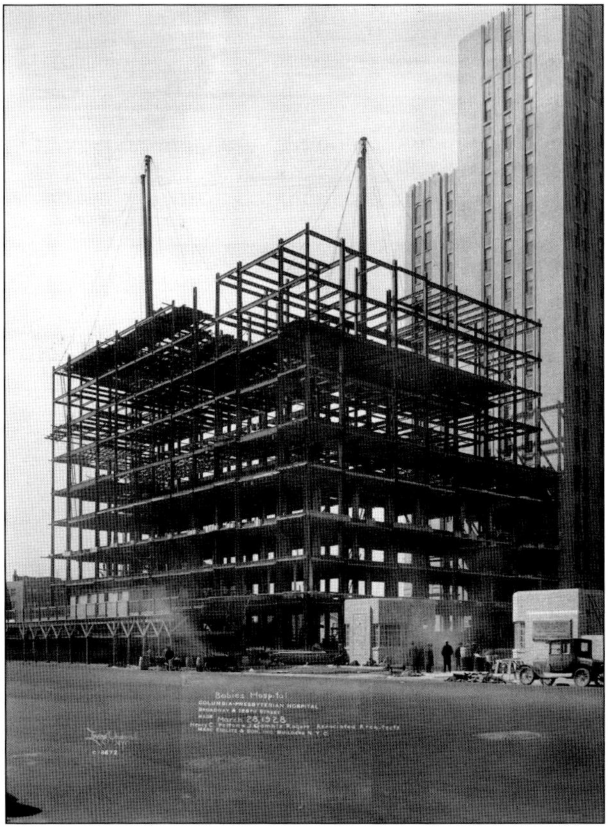

Babies Hospital is seen here under construction at the Columbia-Presbyterian Medical Center in 1928. Although the hospital had affiliated with the medical center in 1925, construction could not begin immediately. A massive fund-raising effort was launched to raise the money needed to build and equip the new structure. The highly successful campaign had many of New York's wealthiest families contributing to the fund, and by early 1928, a total of $1.75 million had been raised. Construction began in January of that year, and by today's standards, the building went up with remarkable speed. The image seen at left, dated March 28, 1928, shows most of the steel frame in place. Only three months later, on June 28 (below), the exterior brickwork was completed. However, finishing the interior took considerably longer, and Babies Hospital only moved to the medical center in June 1929. (Both photographs by Irving Underhill.)

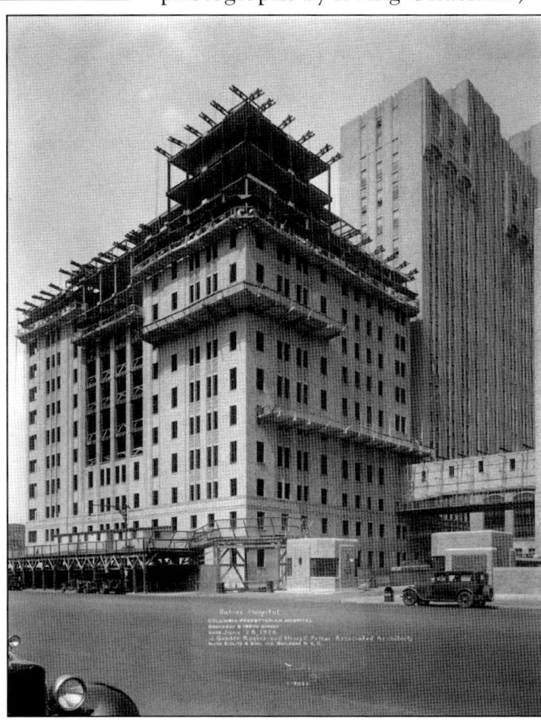

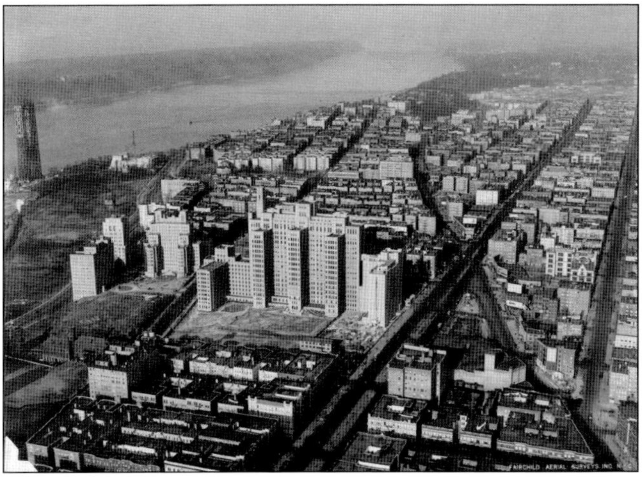

This aerial view from December 1928 shows an almost completed Columbia-Presbyterian Medical Center. From left to right are the School of Nursing's Maxwell Hall, New York State Psychiatric Institute, Neurological Institute, the main complex housing Columbia's medical school and Presbyterian Hospital, and at far right facing Broadway, the Babies Hospital still under construction. Note the tower of the unfinished George Washington Bridge at the upper left. (Photograph by Fairchild Aerial Surveys.)

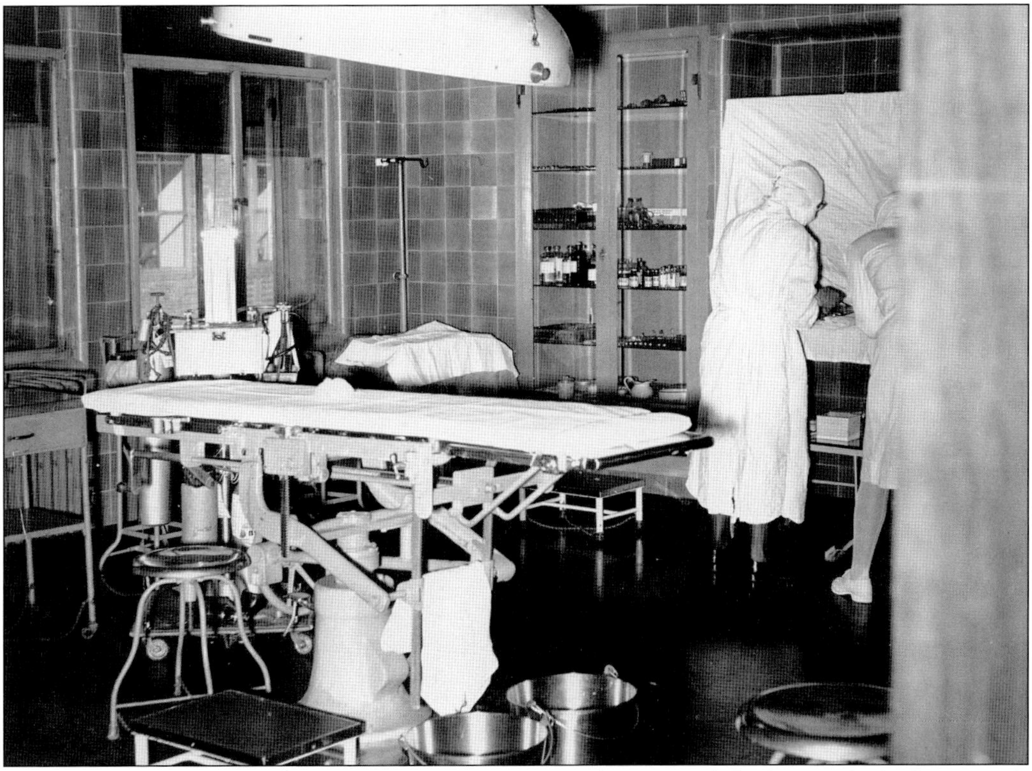

The move to the medical center greatly expanded and improved the hospital's facilities. Beds increased from 55 to 200, allowing Babies Hospital to increase its age limit from three to twelve. New or improved facilities included solaria, private and semiprivate rooms, and according to a fund-raising brochure, "warm rooms for premature babies." Not least of the improvements were up-to-date operating rooms costing $15,000 each, one of which is seen here.

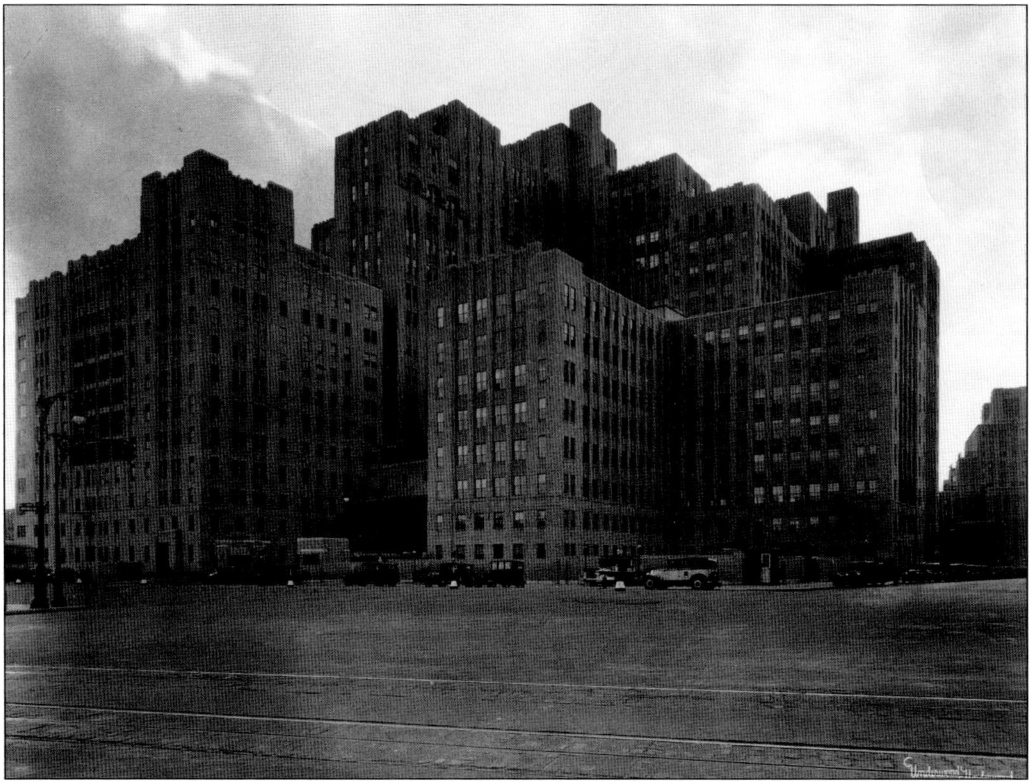

This c. 1930 view of the Columbia-Presbyterian Medical Center looking southwest from the intersection of Broadway and West 168th Street gives an idea of Babies Hospital's placement in the overall complex. It sits at the southeast corner of the campus connected by a bridge to the Vanderbilt Clinic, home of Presbyterian Hospital's out-patient clinic and Columbia's dental school. (Photograph by Underwood & Underwood.)

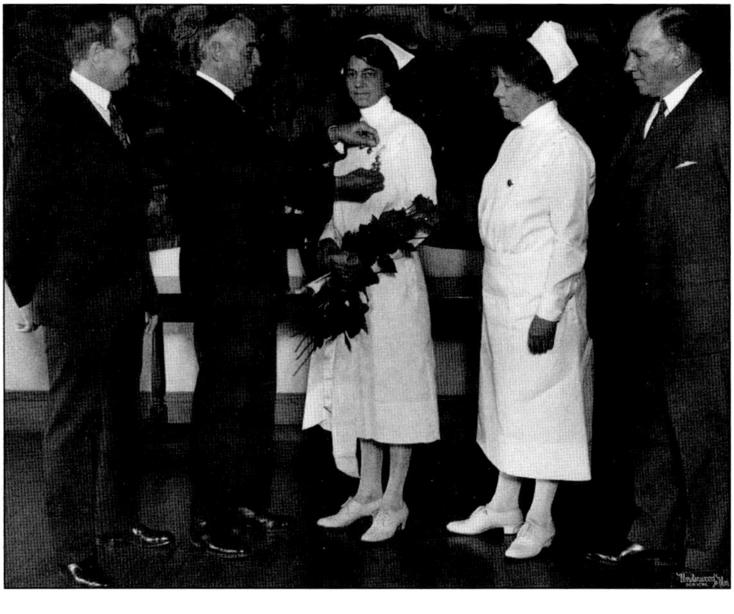

Winifred Kaltenbach, head of nursing at Babies Hospital when the new building opened in 1929, was honored later that year when King Alexander of Yugoslavia bestowed on her the Order of Saint Sava for her previous work as nursing head at the American Hospital of Paris. The king had long been a patron of the hospital and greatly admired Kaltenbach's efforts there. (Photograph by Underwood & Underwood.)

Three

The McIntosh Years

Born in 1894, Rustin McIntosh received a bachelor's degree in 1914 and a medical degree in 1918 from Harvard University. After graduating from medical school, he served as a lieutenant in the Medical Corps of the US Navy with the US Marines until the end of World War I. He completed a residency at the Babies Hospital, worked in a private pediatric practice, had additional training at Johns Hopkins, and returned to Columbia-Presbyterian and the College of Physicians and Surgeons of Columbia University in 1930. He was named Carpentier Professor of Pediatrics in 1931 and became attending pediatrician and director of pediatric service at Babies Hospital, a position he held for almost 30 years.

The McIntosh era fostered a collegial, cohesive atmosphere that engendered clinical and academic excellence. Research flourished, and new child and adolescent-focused subspecialty divisions and sections were created in child neurology, neonatology, radiology, pathology, infectious disease, and hematology-oncology. McIntosh's interests were numerous, and he wrote important papers on varied topics, including congenital malformations, rheumatic fever, and cystic fibrosis.

Dr. McIntosh served as coeditor and coauthor, in collaboration with L. Emmett Holt Jr., son of Luther Emmett Holt, for the 10th edition (1933) through the 13th edition (1962) of *Holt's Diseases of Infancy and Childhood*, the standard textbook in pediatrics.

He served as president of the Society for Pediatric Research in 1934 and the American Pediatric Society in 1953–1954. In 1961, he was awarded the John Howland Award, the highest honor given by the American Pediatric Society. McIntosh married Millicent Carey, who was dean of Barnard College from 1947 to 1952 and president of Barnard College of Columbia University from 1952 to 1962.

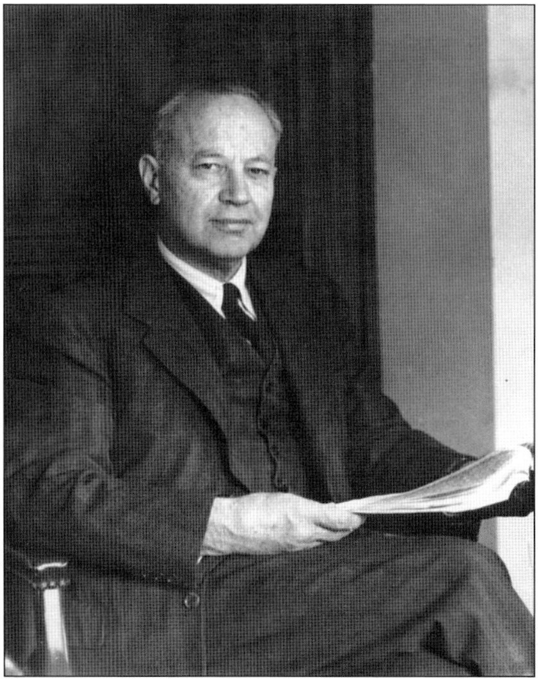

Rustin McIntosh was born in Nebraska in 1894. He attended Harvard University, receiving a bachelor's degree in 1914 and his medical degree in 1918. After graduation, he served in France with the US Marines as a member of the US Navy Medical Corps during World War I. He completed his residency at Babies Hospital and served as chief of the outpatient clinic and as an assistant attending physician. In 1931, he was appointed director of the hospital and chairman of the department of pediatrics at Columbia's College of Physicians and Surgeons. During his almost-30-year tenure, McIntosh brought the hospital to international renown. He established pioneering services in child psychiatry, surgery, radiology, and other disciplines and recruited brilliant researchers such as Hattie Alexander, Dorothy Andersen, and John Caffey. These photographs show him at mid-career (left) and in 1960 (below), the year he retired.

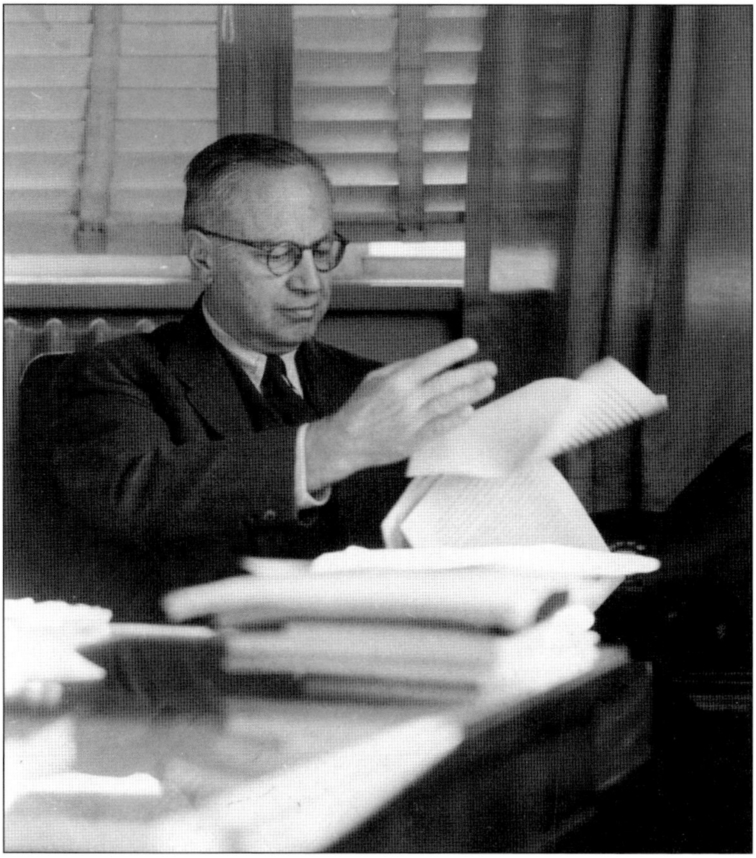

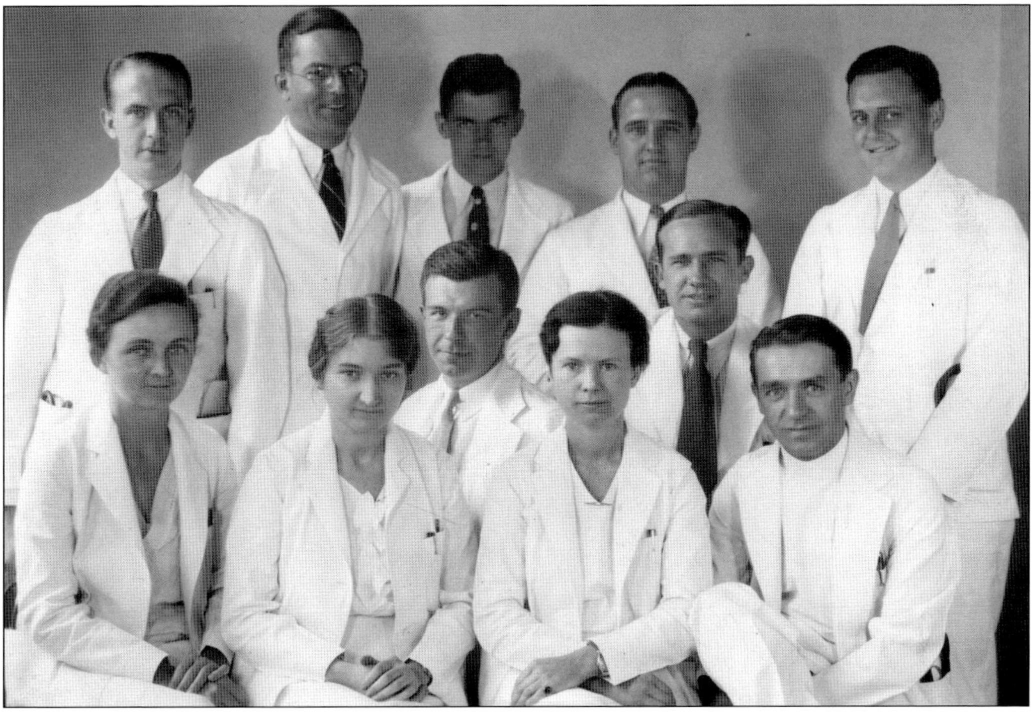

House staff photographs may not change much over the decades, but house staffs do. These two images taken about 60 years apart show the Babies Hospital house staffs for 1932 and 1992–1993. One striking difference is size: the earlier picture (above) has just 11 residents, while the latter one shows 23 (plus 5 faculty). The other is diversity: the 1932 group is entirely white and mostly male. The 1992–1993 class has many more women—a majority in fact—and several minorities. The woman in the first row, second from right, in the 1932 group is Hattie Alexander, who went on to become one of Babies Hospital's most illustrious faculty members, known for her work developing a serum to cure bacterial meningitis. The 1992–1993 image shows department chairman John M. Driscoll at the center.

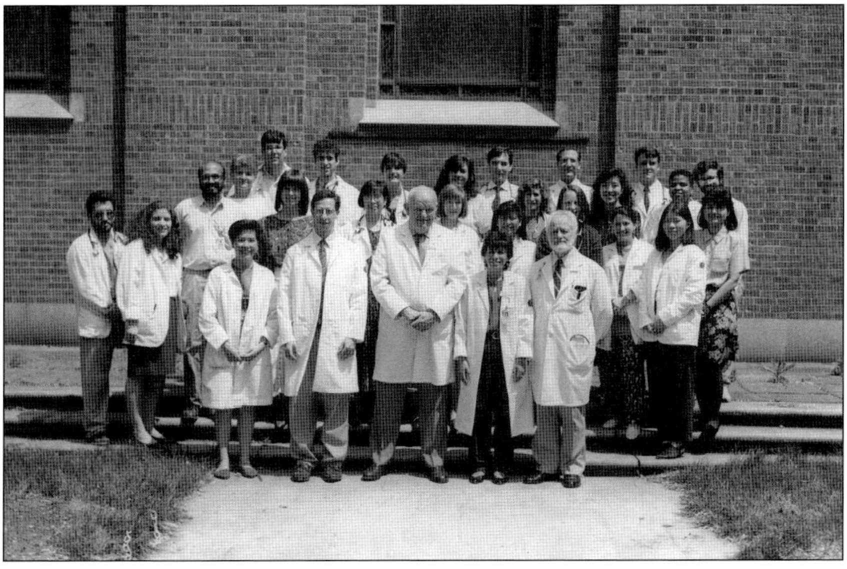

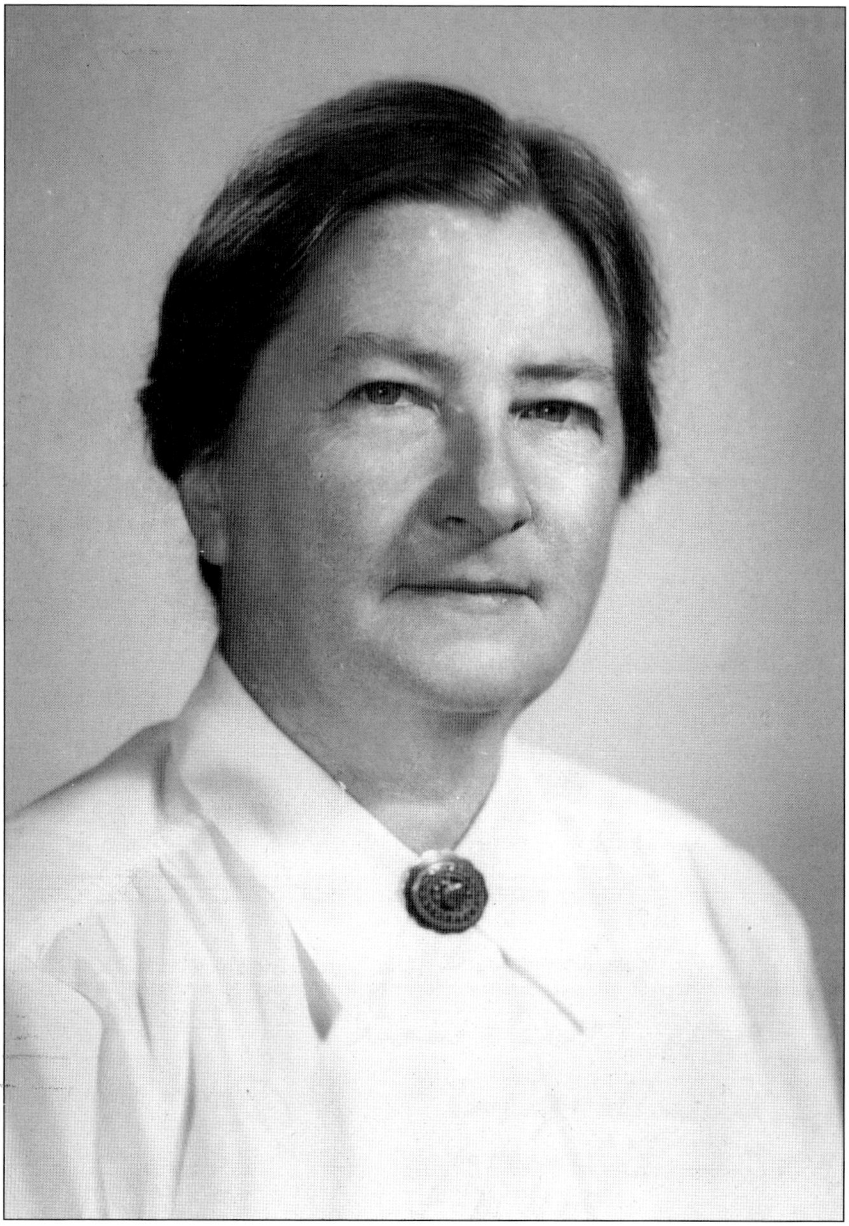

Dorothy Hansine Andersen received her bachelor of arts degree from Mount Holyoke College and a medical degree from Johns Hopkins University. After a residency at Strong Memorial Hospital, University of Rochester, she accepted a position in pathology at Columbia University's medical school in 1929, where she remained for her entire career. Andersen is best known for her description and recognition of cystic fibrosis of the pancreas, which she first described in 1938 in an article in the *American Journal of Diseases of Children*. In 1949, she and colleague Paul di Sant'Agnese developed the sweat test, the first efficient and accurate test for the disease. She was awarded the E. Mead Johnson Award for her recognition of this disease, and in 1952, she was appointed chief of pathology at the Babies Hospital, a position she held until her death in 1963. She served as a consultant to the Armed Forces Institute of Pathology during World War II. Among her many honors are the Elizabeth Blackwell Award and induction into the Women's Hall of Fame in 2001.

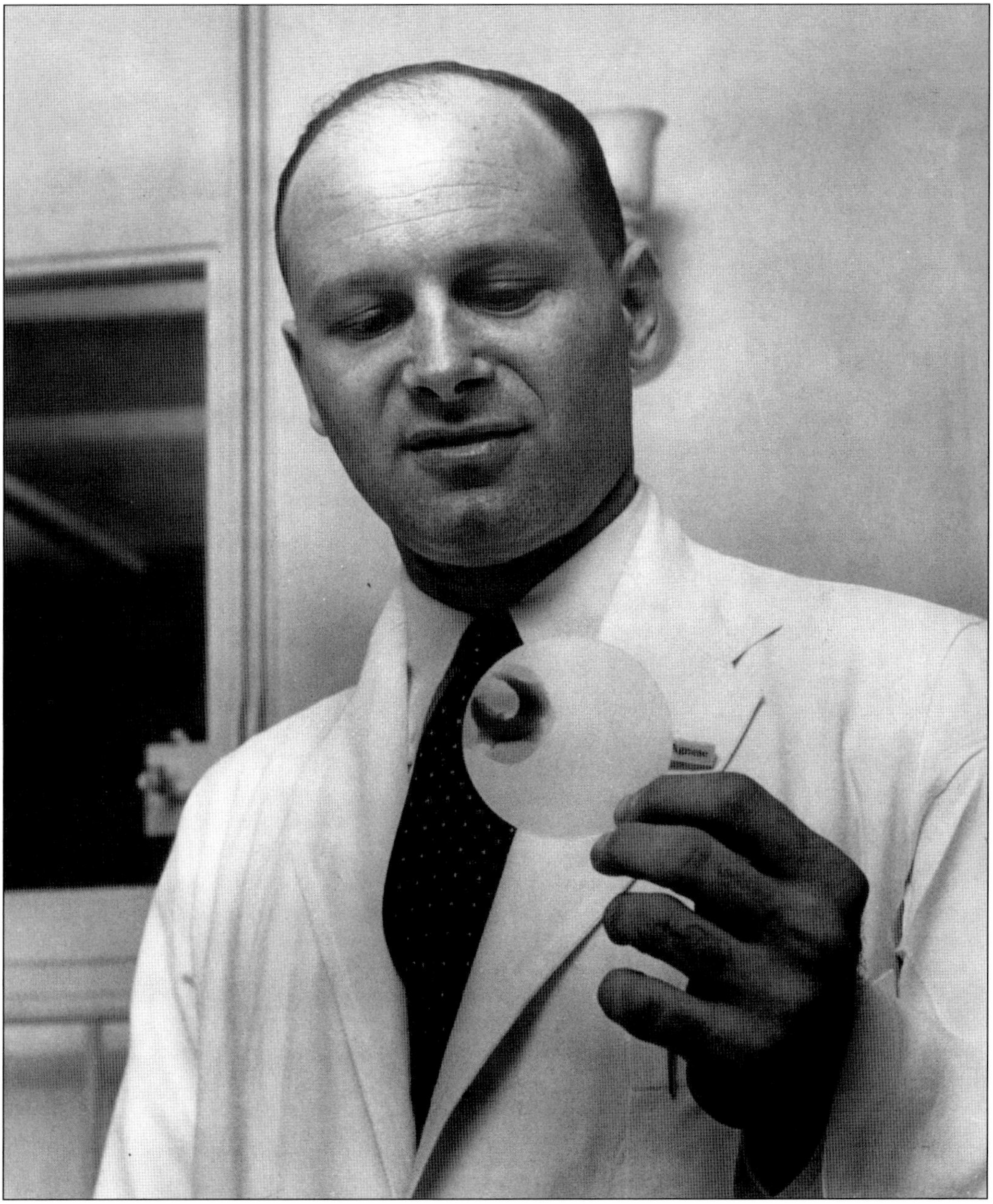

A native of Italy, Dr. Paul di Sant'Agnese received his medical degree from the University of Rome before immigrating to the United States. At Columbia, he earned a doctor of medical science degree in 1948 and became a member of the department of pathology at Babies Hospital. Building on the work of Dorothy Andersen, di Sant'Agnese observed during a 1949 heat wave that infants suffering from cystic fibrosis were at special risk for dehydration. The recognition of abnormalities in the salt content of sweat led to the development of the sweat test as the primary method of diagnosing cystic fibrosis. This remains the cornerstone of the diagnosis of the disease and opened up areas of research that ultimately helped to identify the basic defect involved in cystic fibrosis. He was a founder of the Cystic Fibrosis Foundation and, as a physician and researcher, was one of the first clinicians to devote his life to understanding and conquering this disease.

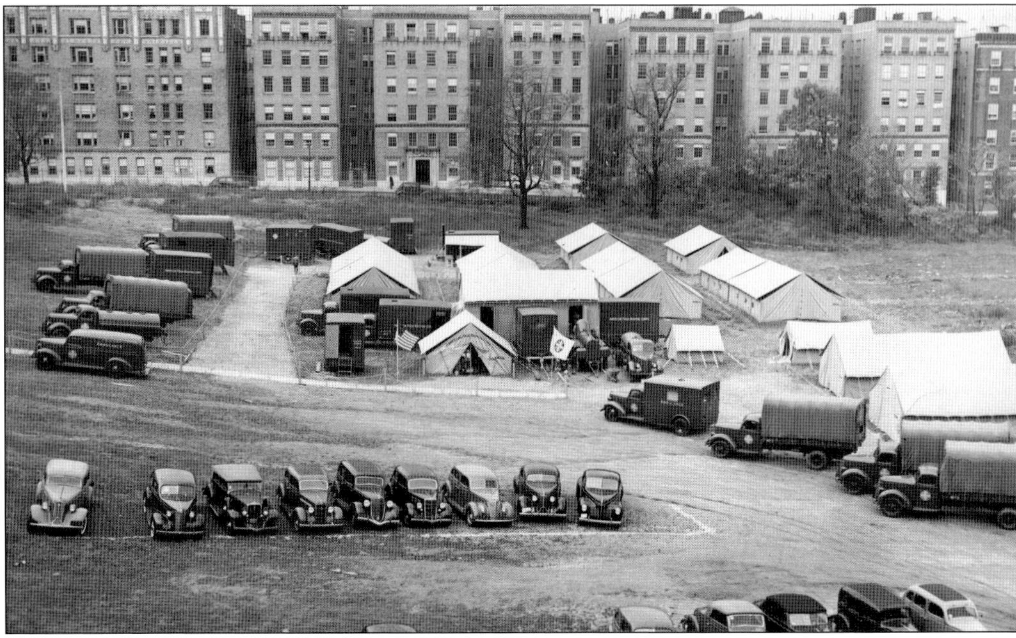

Babies Hospital answered its country's call when the United States entered World War II in 1941. At least 65 hospital personnel served in overseas military hospitals. Many were members of US General Hospital No. 2, generally called "2nd General" and largely staffed by Columbia-Presbyterian Medical Center physicians and nurses. Planning had begun well before the outbreak of hostilities, allowing a test run of the hospital on the grounds of the campus in 1942 (above). After training at Fort Meade, Maryland, in July 1942, the more than 100 men and women of the 2nd General reached Oxford, England, their base for the next two years. Several weeks after D-Day, they were stationed at Lison in Normandy, just behind the front. Below, a wounded soldier is placed in an ambulance somewhere in France in 1944.

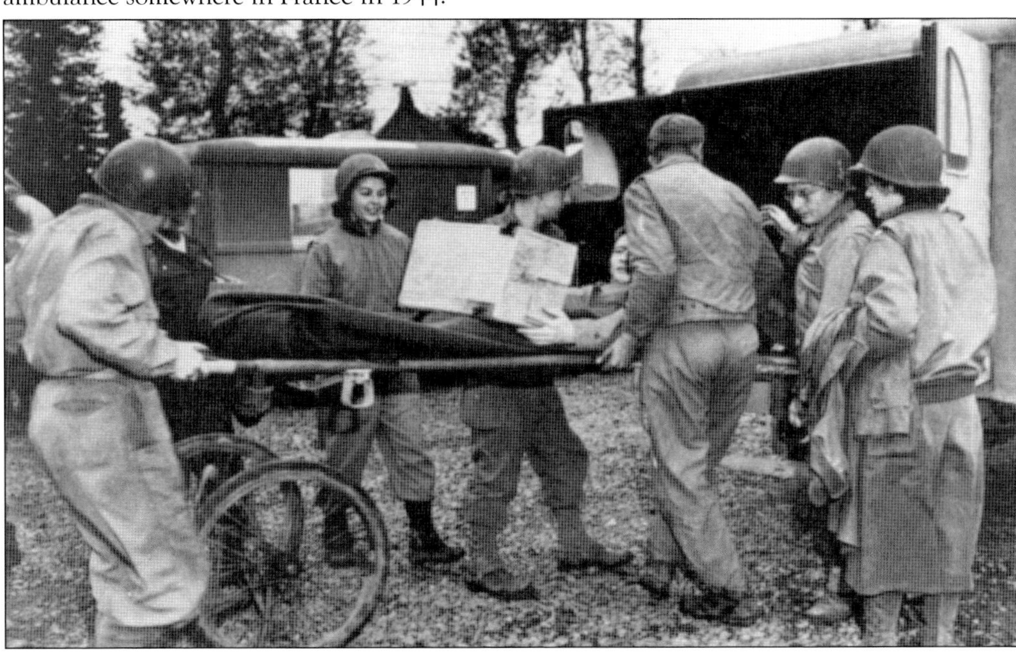

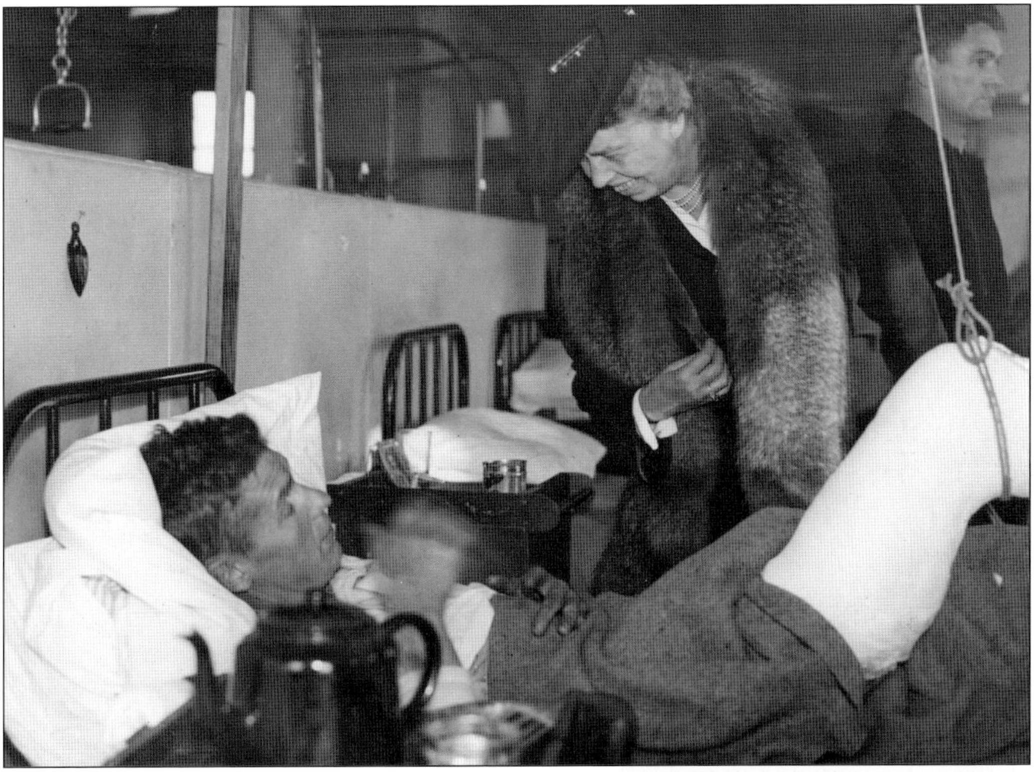

The two years 2nd General spent in Oxford were relatively normal for wartime. Though rationing and air raids were ever-present, there were plenty of diversions in the ancient university town. Chief among them were numerous visits from celebrities. Indefatigable First Lady Eleanor Roosevelt is seen here comforting a soldier at 2nd General—one of the dozens of visits she made to military hospitals on several fronts during the war.

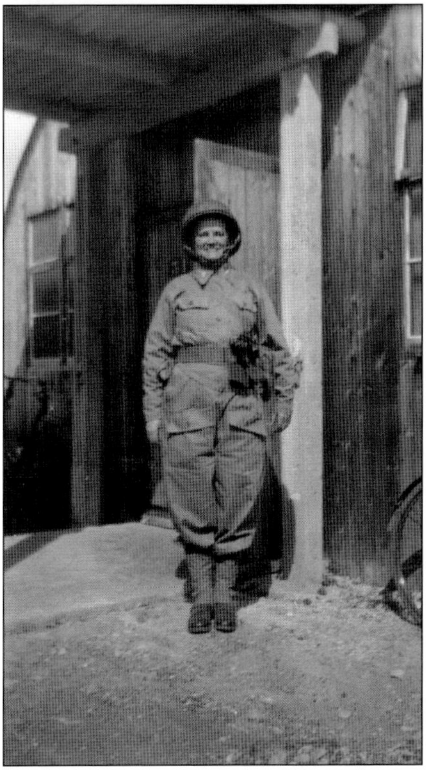

Arrayed in battle gear, Marjorie Peto, chief nurse of 2nd General, is seen here probably in France. Peto was responsible for managing nursing care at the hospital and in charge of about 50 nurses. In 1946, she became director of nursing at Babies Hospital, a position she held for 23 years, and she still found time to write a war memoir, *Women Were Not Expected*.

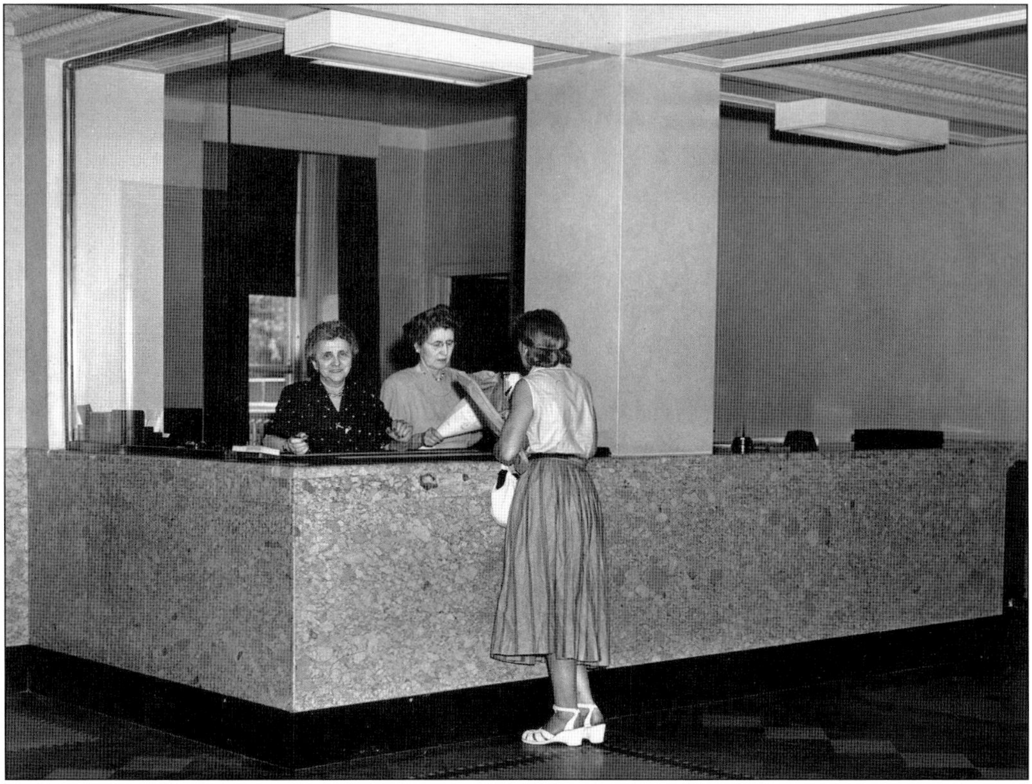

The immediate post–World War II era did not see many infrastructure changes at Babies Hospital. However, in 1950–1951, the doctors' private patients practice suite was renovated to include a new waiting room, and the information/reception desk seen here was constructed. That only one person is at the desk would no doubt amaze current hospital reception staff. (Photograph by Lawrence G. Heinrich.)

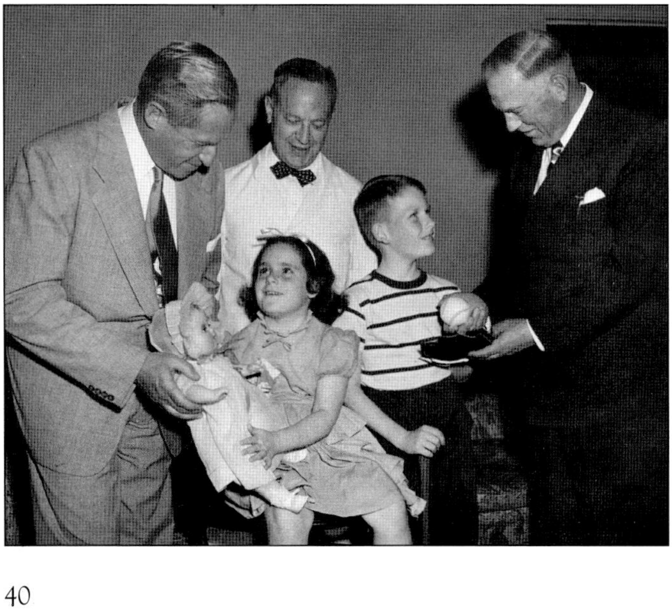

Two patients, Michele Griffin and her brother Robert Griffin, admitted for tonsillectomies on June 7, 1950, are greeted with presents in honor of being medical center patients number 999,999 (Robert) and 1 million (Michele). Seen behind them are, from left to right, Robert W. Dowling, campaign chairman, Greater New York Fund; Dr. Rustin D. McIntosh, director, Babies Hospital; and Charles P. Cooper, Presbyterian Hospital president. (Photograph by Acme Newspictures.)

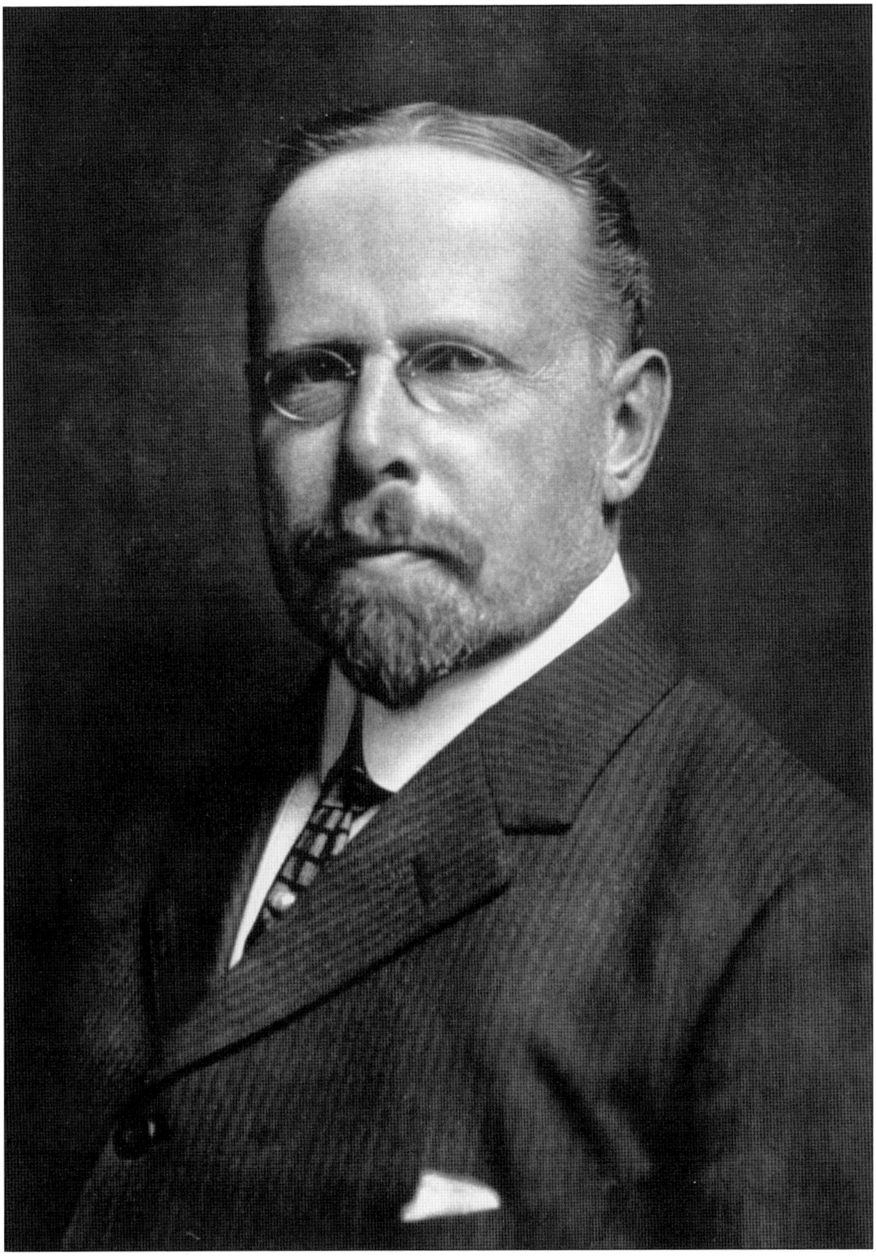

Founded in the early 20th century by renowned neurologist Dr. Bernard Sachs, the Division of Child Neurology at Columbia's Neurological Institute was the first service in the nation focused solely on the distinct neurological needs of children and their developing nervous systems. Dr. Sachs had many notable achievements including his textbook, *Nervous Diseases of Children* (1895), and a popular manual on childrearing, *The Normal Child* (1926), as well as contributing to the classification of cerebral palsy (1926). However, he is probably best remembered for Tay-Sachs disease, a genetic disorder he described with his colleague, Warren Tay, an English ophthalmologist. In 1881, Dr. Tay first described the red spot on the retina of the eye characteristic of this rare disease, while Dr. Sachs provided a more comprehensive description and in 1887 noted its higher occurrence in Ashkenazi Jews from Eastern Europe. (National Library of Medicine.)

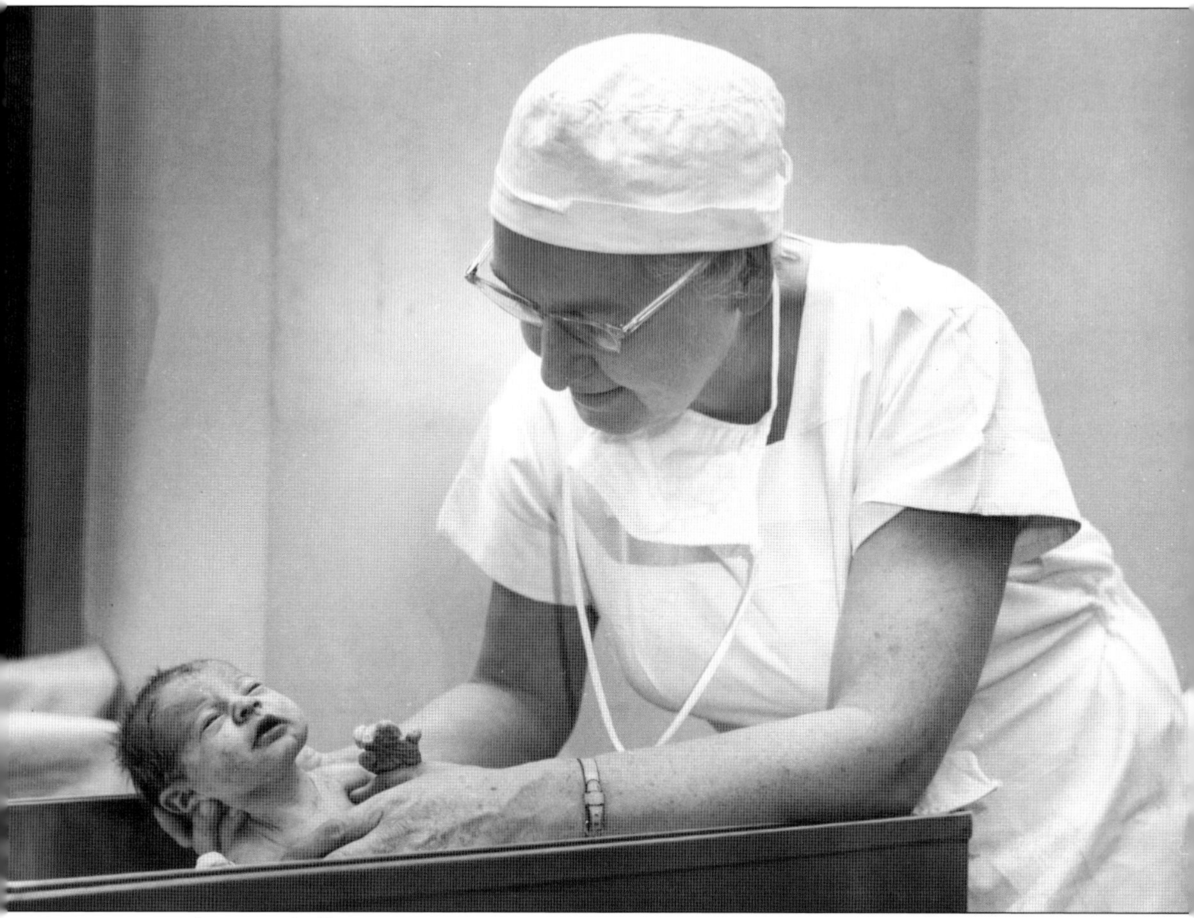

One of the many brilliant women on the Columbia medical school faculty in the mid-20th century, Virginia Apgar graduated from the College of Physicians and Surgeons in 1933 and completed a residency in surgery at Columbia-Presbyterian Medical Center in 1937. As an anesthesiologist, she was the first woman named chief of a subspecialty division at the medical center and, in 1949, became the first woman to become a full tenured professor at the College of Physicians and Surgeons. Apgar studied infant mortality within the first 24 hours of life and developed a standardized scoring system to assess infant health at 1 minute and 5 minutes after birth. Newborns are assigned a grade—0, 1, or 2—for the following parameters: heart rate, respiration, color, muscle tone, and irritability. The Apgar score is still used today for reporting the status of the newborn infant immediately after birth. Besides her professional interests, Apgar enjoyed fishing, golf, and stamp collecting. An excellent violist, she was known for making her own instruments. (Photograph by Elizabeth Wilcox.)

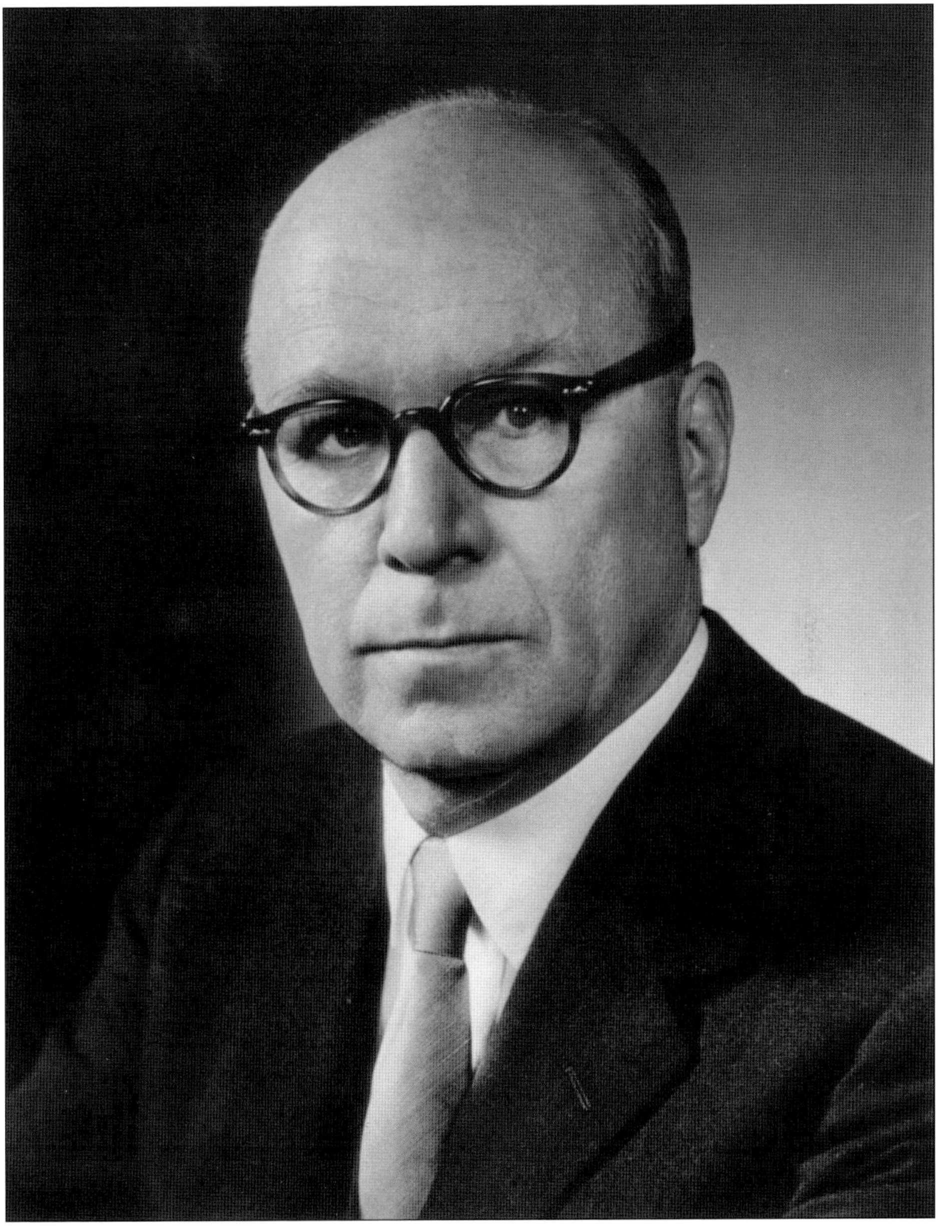

Dr. Algernon Reese graduated from Davidson College and the Harvard University Medical School. After laying the foundation for his career in ophthalmic pathology by studying with Frederick Verhoef in Boston and Ernest Fuchs in Vienna, Reese was on the staff of the New York Eye and Ear Clinic from 1923 to 1927. He had a brief tenure at Cornell's medical school before coming to Columbia University to join its Department of Ophthalmology in 1931. He spent more than 50 years at the university caring for patients with diseases of the eye. He was the founder of the field of ophthalmic oncology; his primary contribution to ophthalmological medicine was in the treatment of retinoblastoma, a malignant eye tumor in children. He established the guidelines for diagnosis and treatment of the ailment and set up the first clinic for its patients. Reese developed the Reese-Ellsworth classification of retinoblastoma to predict a patient's prognosis after treatment with radiation. (National Library of Medicine.)

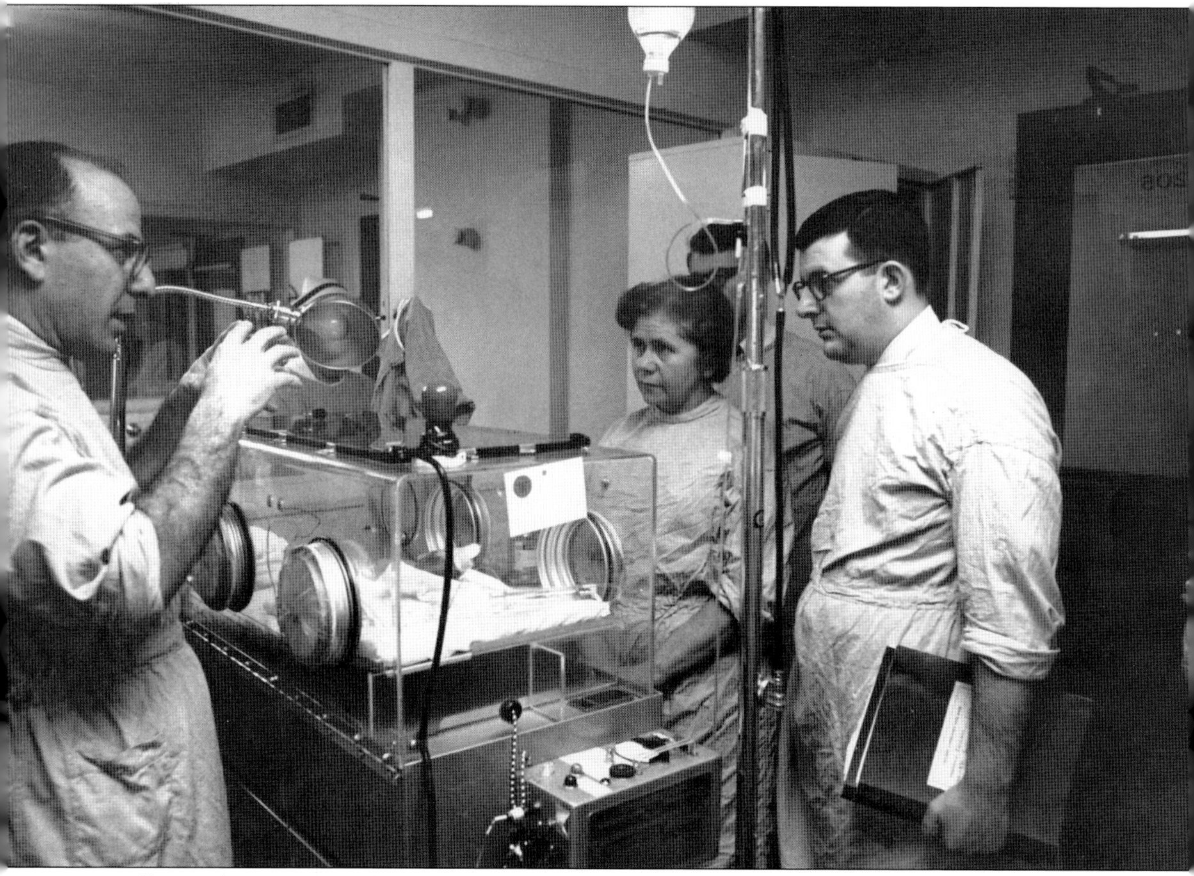

William Silverman completed undergraduate studies at the University of California, Los Angeles, and earned a medical degree from the University of California, San Francisco. After completion of a pediatric residency at the Babies Hospital, Columbia-Presbyterian Medical Center, he remained on the faculty and became the first director of the neonatal intensive care unit in 1946. Silverman's research contributed to the finding that retrolental fibroplasia, now known as retinopathy of prematurity, was secondary to high oxygen concentrations. His research was grounded by the belief that scientific evidence must guide clinical decision making, and he is considered the father of evidence-based medicine. Silverman urged physicians to address considerations like the quality of life in formulating medical treatment plans, especially in the management of premature infants. Silverman was adamant that strong scientific evidence must guide medical decision making, and it has been said that he was "clearly the pioneer" in evidence-based medicine. In this photograph, Silverman, on the left, discusses the management of a patient in the Babies Hospital neonatal intensive care unit with two unidentified members of house staff. (Photograph by Elizabeth Wilcox.)

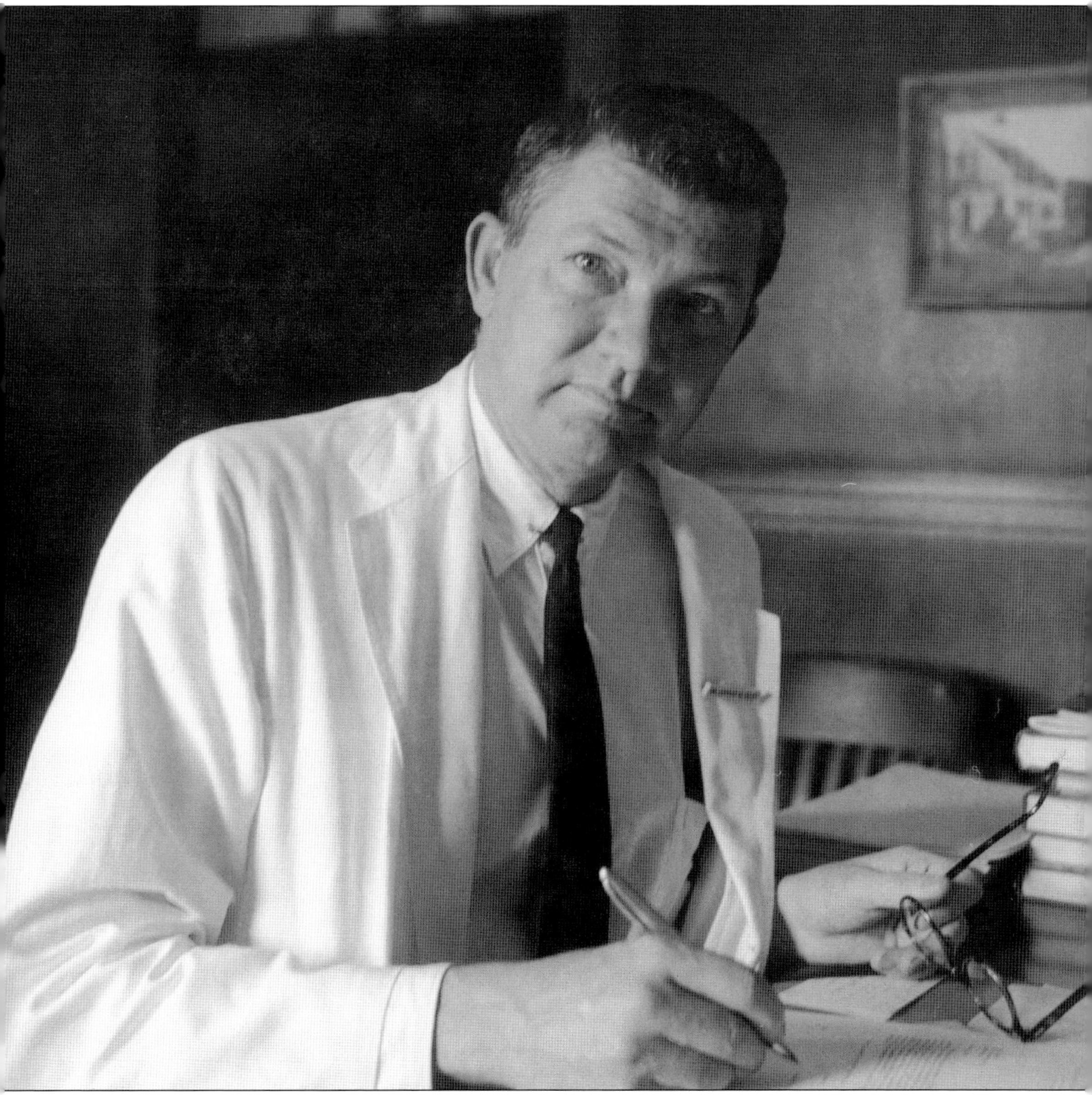

Conrad M. Riley, seen here in 1959, was educated at Yale (AB, 1934) and Harvard (MD, 1938) and served residencies at both Babies and Boston Children's Hospitals. After wartime service in the US Navy, Riley joined Babies Hospital in 1946. There, his main research interest was in nephrosis, and he and Dr. Alice Davis established a clinic that helped advance understanding of the disease. However, Riley is best known as a codiscoverer of a completely different ailment. In 1949, he and his colleague Dr. Richard L. Day identified a complex disease most commonly found in Jewish children of Ashkenazi descent. The symptoms included seizures, insensitivity to pain, vomiting, extremes in blood pressure, inability to produce tears, and delay in puberty. The disorder, known as Riley-Day syndrome, is caused by a defective gene inherited from both parents and can lead to death before the age of 20. Riley left Babies Hospital in 1960 to become a professor of preventive medicine at the University of Colorado's medical school. (Photograph by Elizabeth Wilcox.)

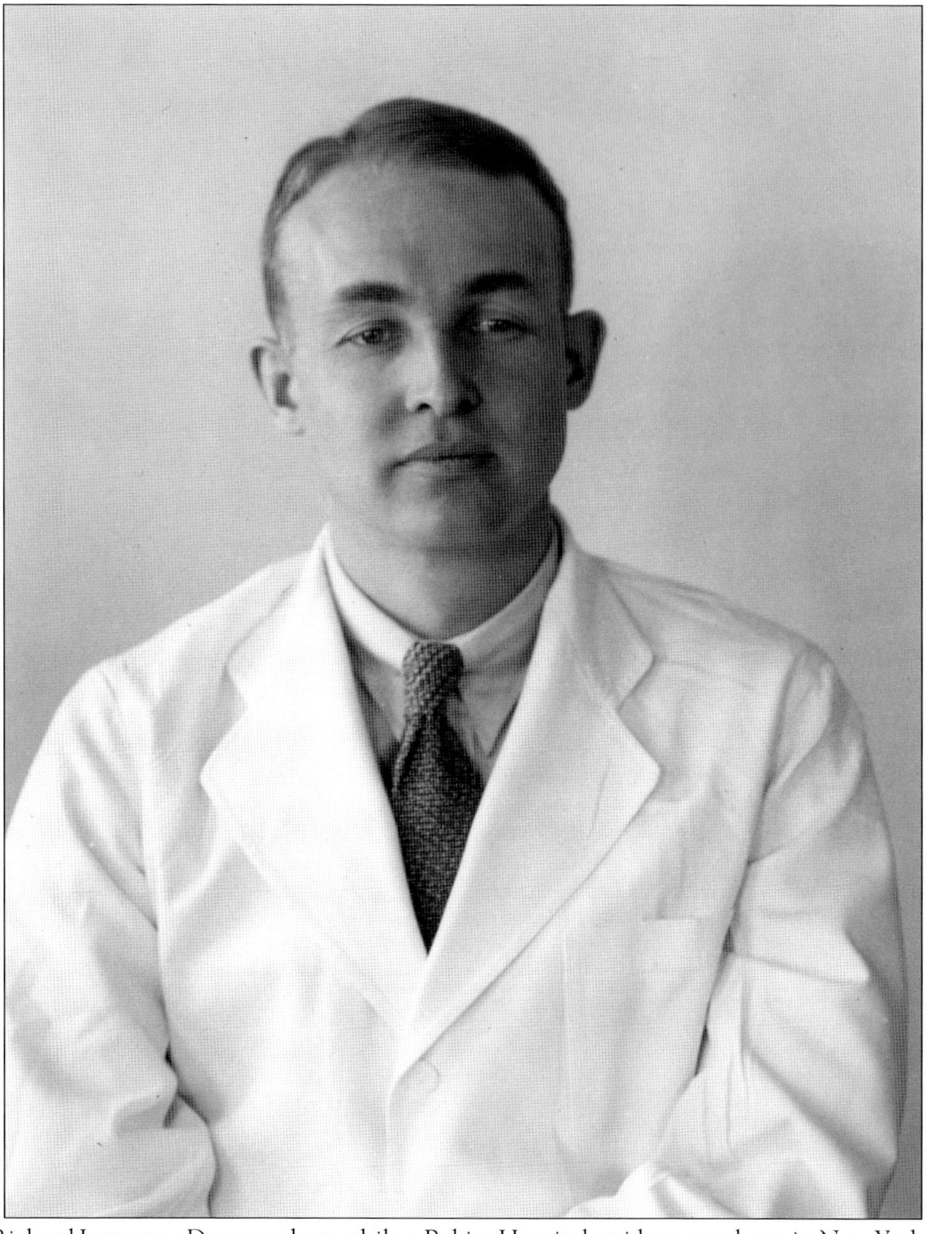

Dr. Richard Lawrence Day, seen here while a Babies Hospital resident, was born in New York City in 1905. He received both his undergraduate and medical degrees from Harvard University. In 1933, Day began his residency training at the Babies Hospital, and in 1935, he joined the faculty of the department of pediatrics at the College of Physicians and Surgeons, Columbia University. Day established the first unit for premature infants in the nation at Babies Hospital in 1949. He was recognized for his studies of the mechanism controlling the body temperature of premature babies and for his discovery that the yellow pigment bilirubin damaged the extrapyramidal nuclei of the infant brain. He left Columbia in 1953, and for the next 12 years, he served successively as chairman of the pediatric departments at State University of New York's Downstate Medical Center and the University of Pittsburgh. He would later serve as the medical director of Planned Parenthood International.

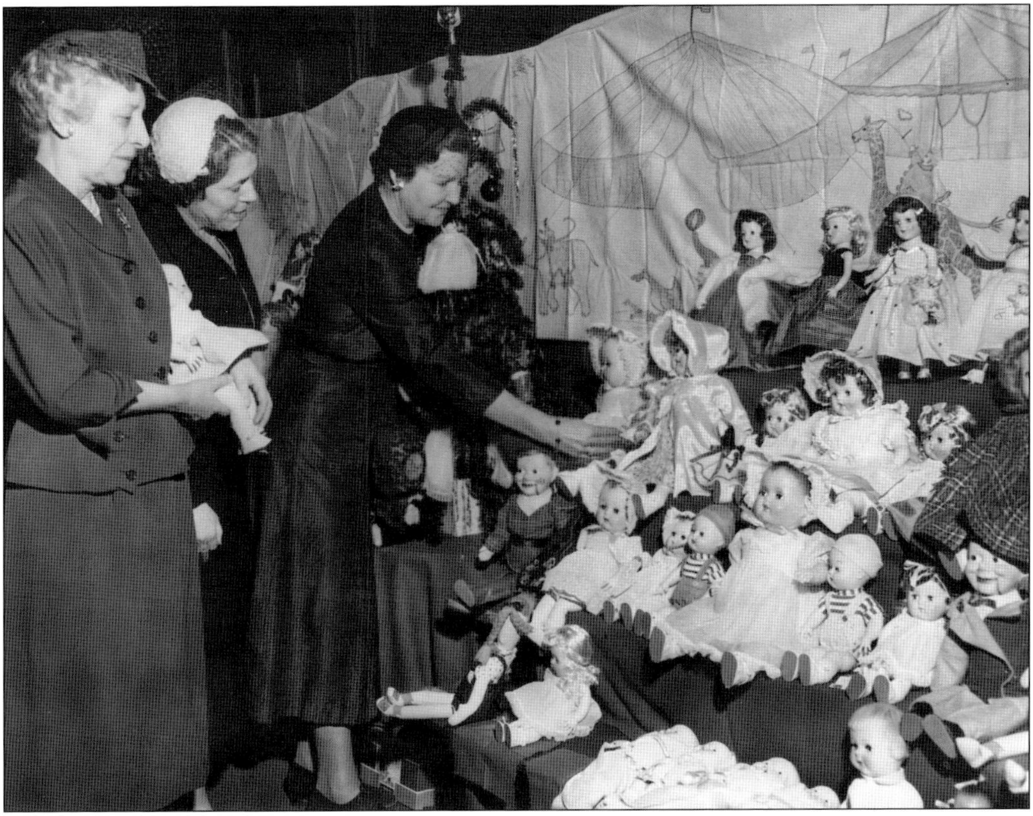

The Babies Hospital Board of Women Managers, originally known as the Board of Lady Managers, was founded along with the hospital in 1887 and supported it through a variety of endeavors both as volunteers and fund-raisers. Here, several board members look at the dolls donated for the annual Dolls' Tea Party in 1952. The dolls were then presented to patients on Christmas Day. (Photograph by Manny Warman.)

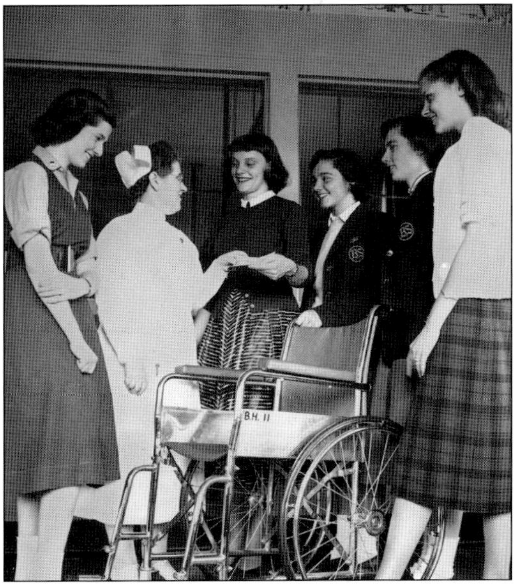

Babies Hospital has always gratefully accepted gifts large and small. In May 1953, Cecily Slade, vice president of the senior class at Manhattan's Brearley School, presents a class gift of $75 for the purchase of a wheelchair like the one shown here. Accepting it on behalf of the hospital is Elna Saamenen, the fourth-floor head nurse. Surrounding her are other members of the Brearley class committee. (Photograph by Manny Warman.)

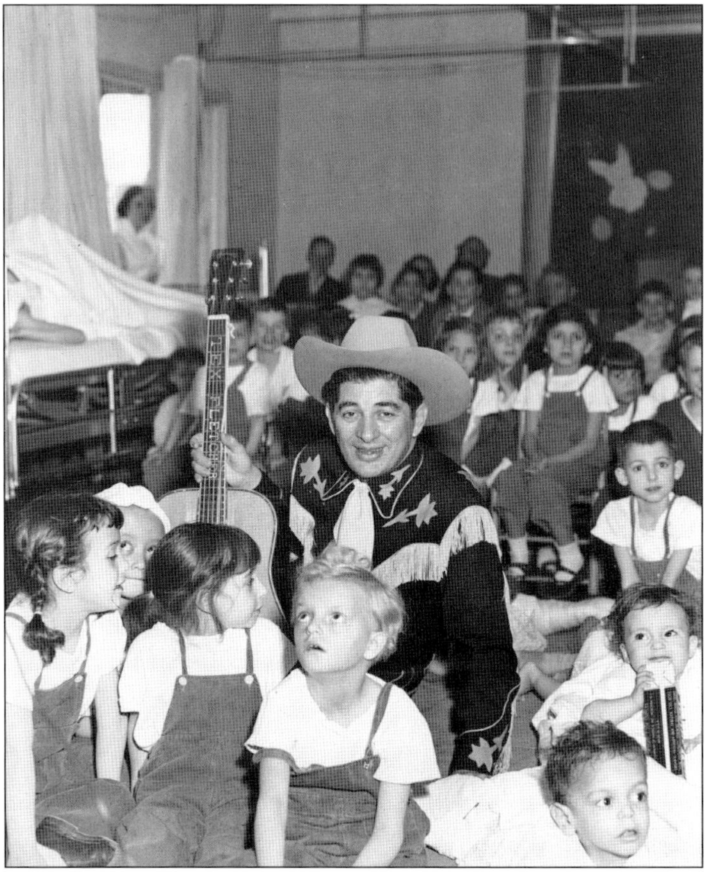

Celebrities from the worlds of sports, television, movies, and music have all made the trek to Babies Hospital to entertain patients. At left, Tex Fletcher, cowboy star of the *Tootsie Hippodrome* television show, is seen with children at an Easter party held on the fifth floor of the hospital in 1953. Fletcher was one of the country's biggest "cowboy singers" of the mid-20th century. Below, Morris the Cat, spokescat for a leading cat food brand, appears at the hospital in 1986. While the child seems interested in being so close to a celebrity feline, Morris, true to form, remains finicky. (Left, photograph by William H. Banks.)

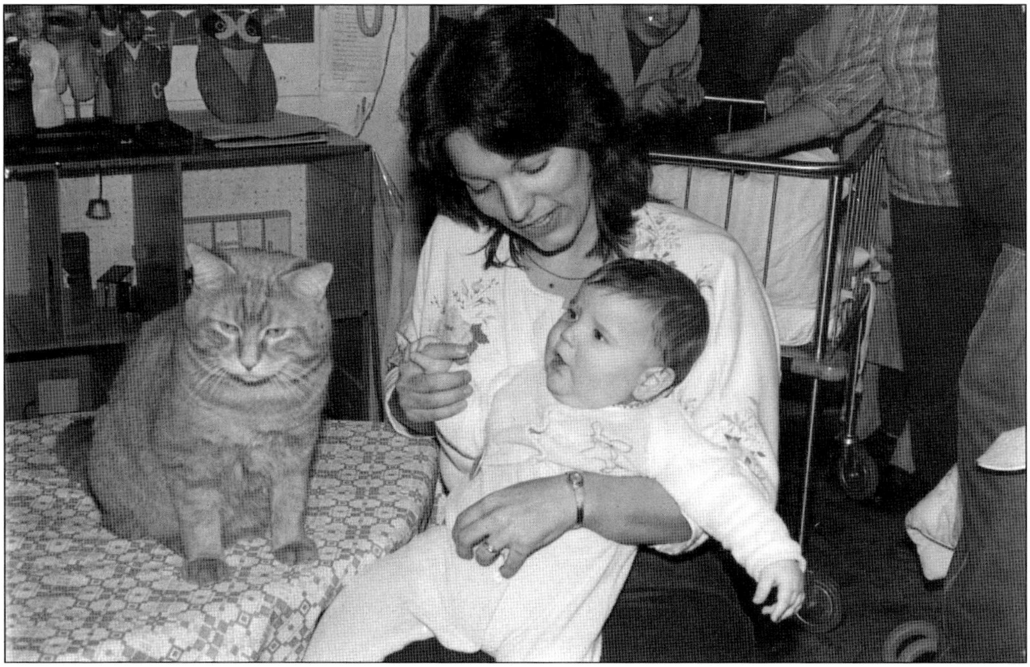

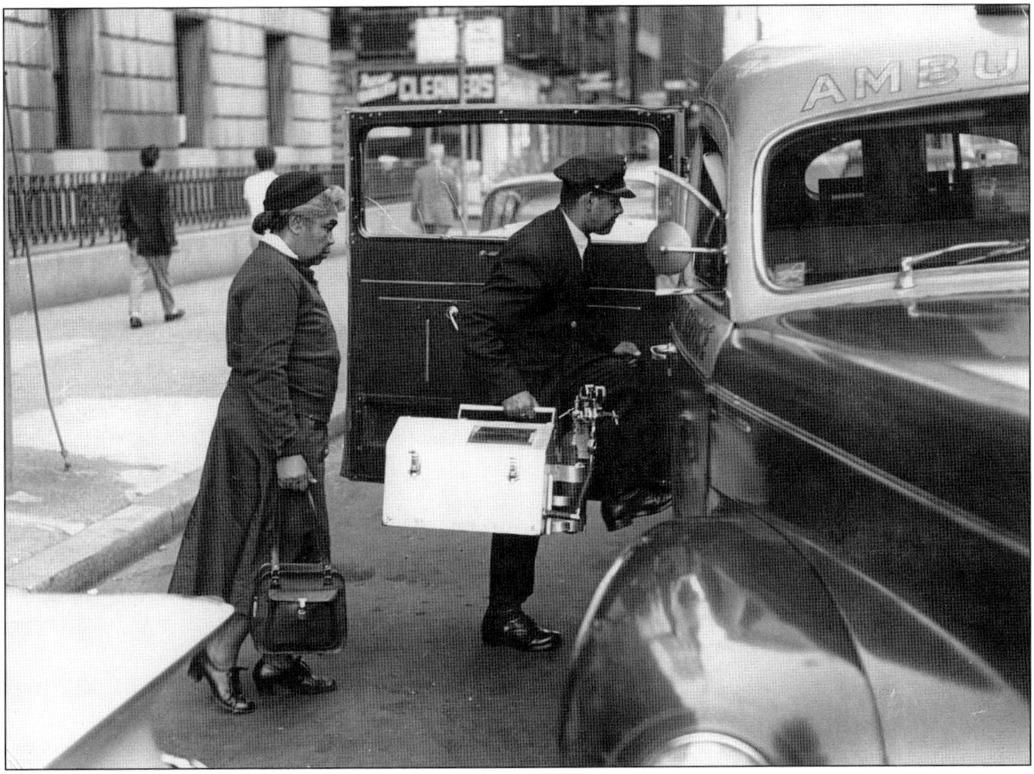

A matron and driver from the New York City Premature Infant Transport program bring their tiny patient to Babies Hospital in 1954. That year, the hospital's premature nursery, founded in 1949, admitted its 1,000th infant. The technology of premature care was still primitive in the 1950s: the portable incubator held by the driver is a remodeled pet carrier.

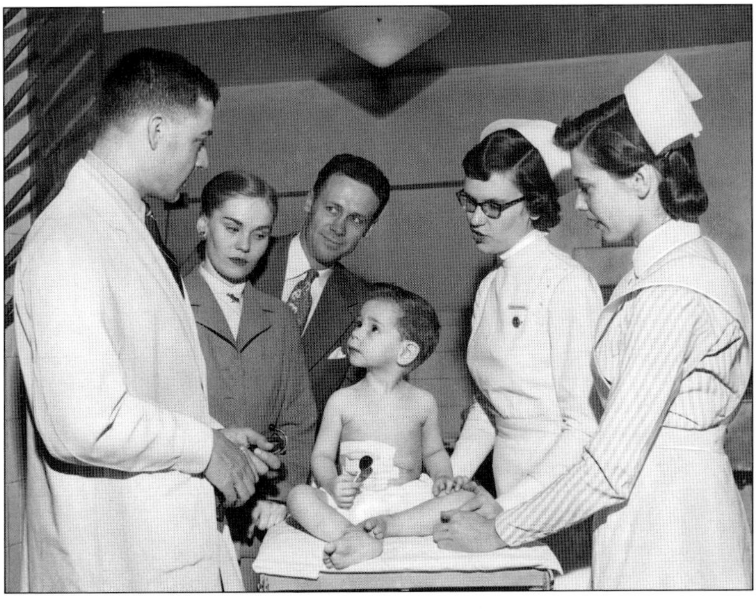

This little boy does not seem to be intimidated by the concerned adults surrounding him in 1954. At left is Dr. William Bauman, then chief of pediatrics at the medical center's Vanderbilt Clinic. A 1947 graduate of Columbia's College of Physicians and Surgeons, Bauman joined Babies Hospital in 1948 as a resident and spent his entire career there.

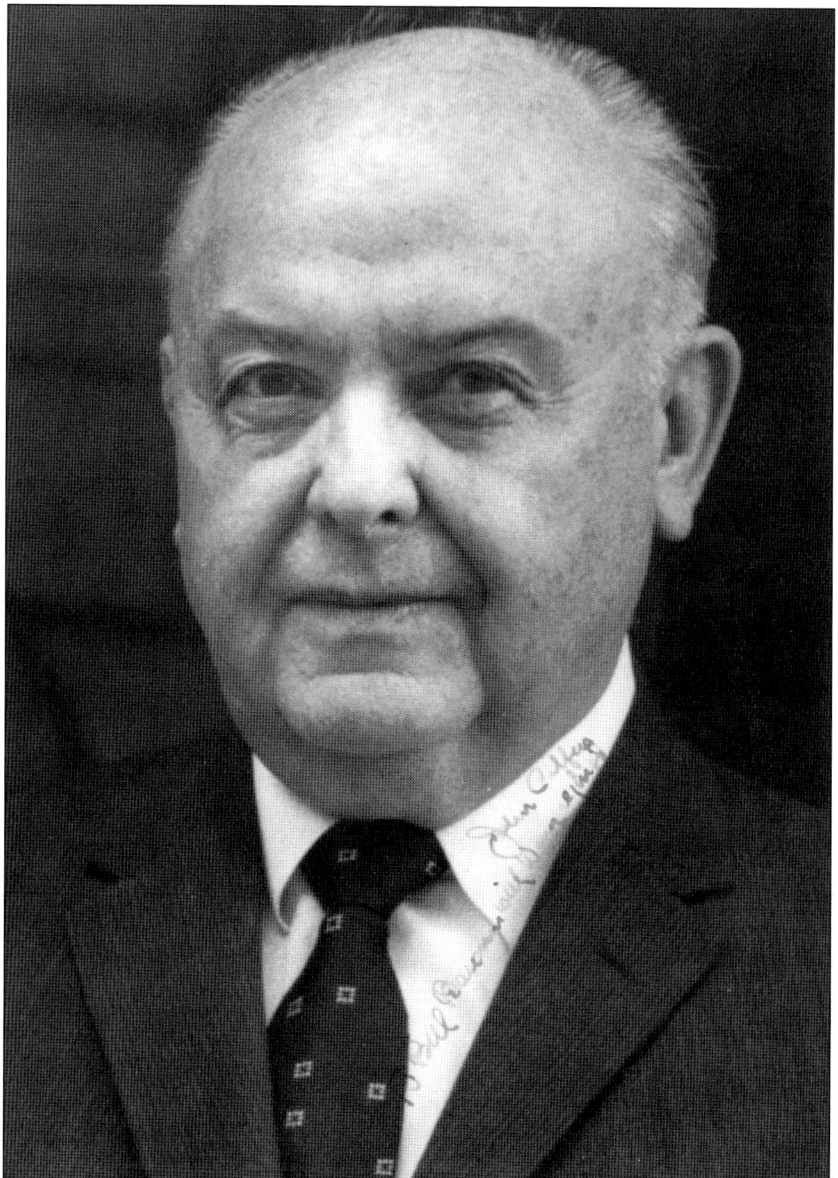

John Caffey was born in 1895 in Utah, the same year Wilhelm Conrad Röntgen discovered x-rays. He received both his undergraduate and medical degrees from the University of Michigan and interned at Barnes Hospital in St. Louis, Missouri. Caffey completed a residency in pediatrics at Babies Hospital, where he remained on the faculty for his entire career. He was one of the first pediatric radiologists in North America after having taught himself normal pediatric radiology. Caffey considered radiology to be the fifth component of physical examination with the belief it represented an internal inspection of the body's anatomy. He wrote many scholarly articles, some of which were seminal, including a description of infantile cortical hyperostosis, now known as Caffey disease. His observations on the presence of fractures in the long bones of infants suffering from subdural hematomas led to the recognition of battered child syndrome. In 1945, he published the voluminous textbook *Pediatric X-Ray Diagnosis*. He was the first director of pediatric radiology at the Babies Hospital and a founding member of the Society for Pediatric Radiology.

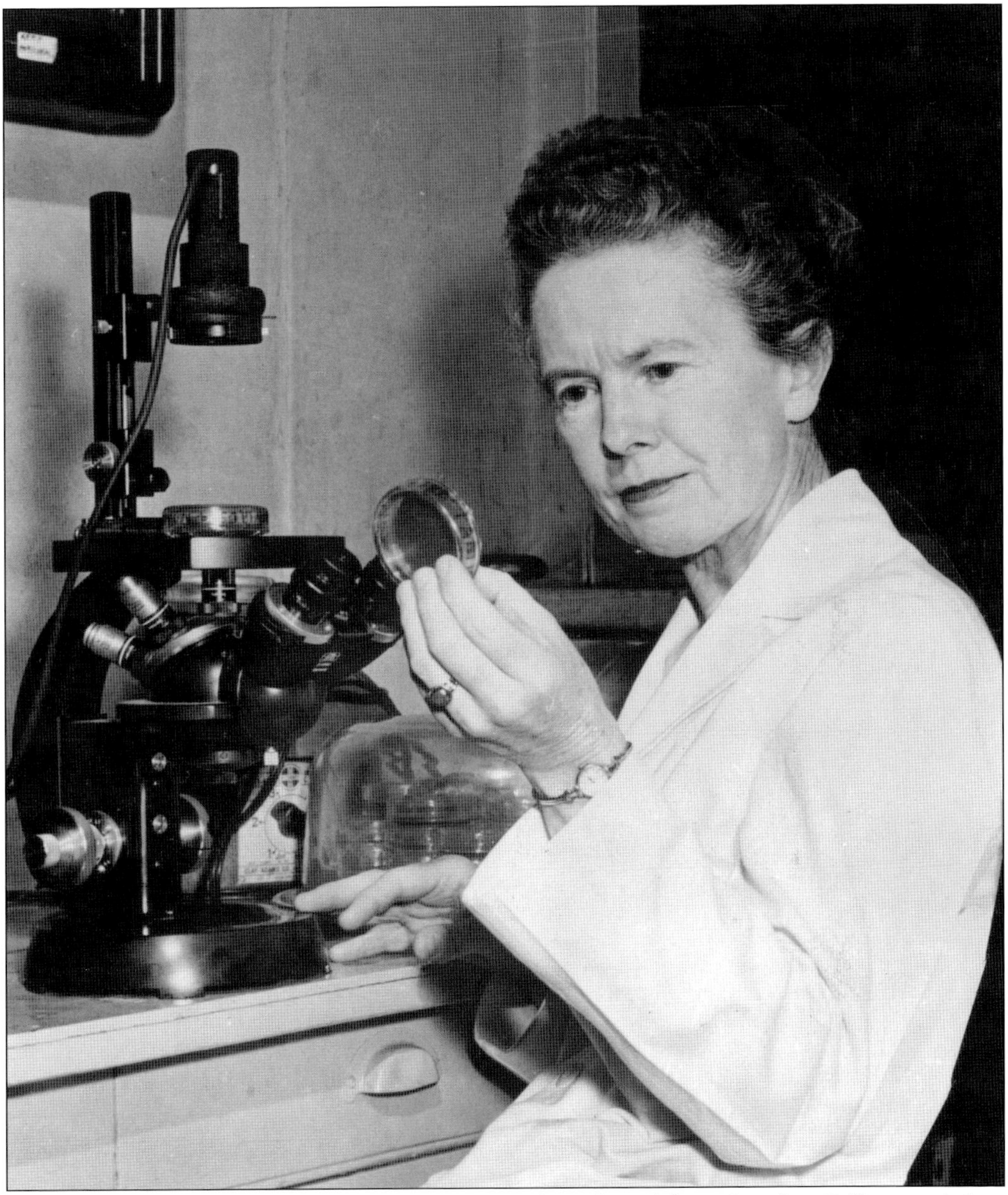

Hattie Alexander was born in Baltimore, Maryland, graduated from Goucher College, and then enrolled at Johns Hopkins University School of Medicine, where she received her medical degree. In 1932, she became an instructor and researcher in the Department of Pediatrics at the Babies Hospital, Columbia-Presbyterian Medical Center, where she spent her entire professional career. In the early 1940s, Alexander began researching *Haemophilus influenzae* (Hib), at the time an almost invariably fatal disease in infants and young children. She developed the first effective treatment for Hib by combining antiserum therapy with sulfa drugs. Alexander subsequently studied the effect of antibiotics on Hib, finding streptomycin to be highly effective. The combined use of the antiserum, sulfa drugs, and antibiotics significantly lowered the mortality rate from Hib. Hattie Alexander was elected president of the American Pediatric Society, the first woman to occupy this position. Outside of work, Alexander was fond of racing her speedboat on Long Island Sound.

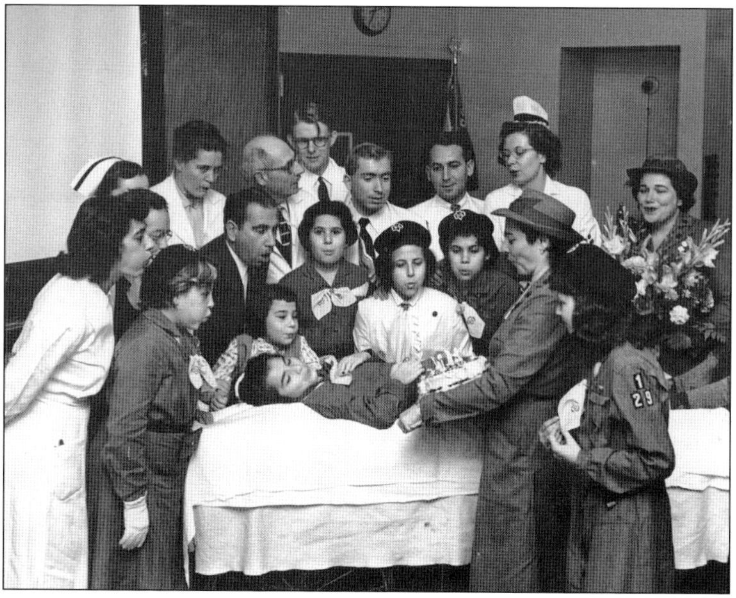

Babies Hospital patient Esther Katzen celebrates her 11th birthday with induction into Girl Scout Troop 129 in November 1954. Esther had helped found the troop several months before but had not yet been enrolled when she contracted polio. Her mother, the troop's leader, presents Esther with her Girl Scout pin and a birthday cake while fellow troop members and the doctors, nurses, and physical therapists caring for her look on.

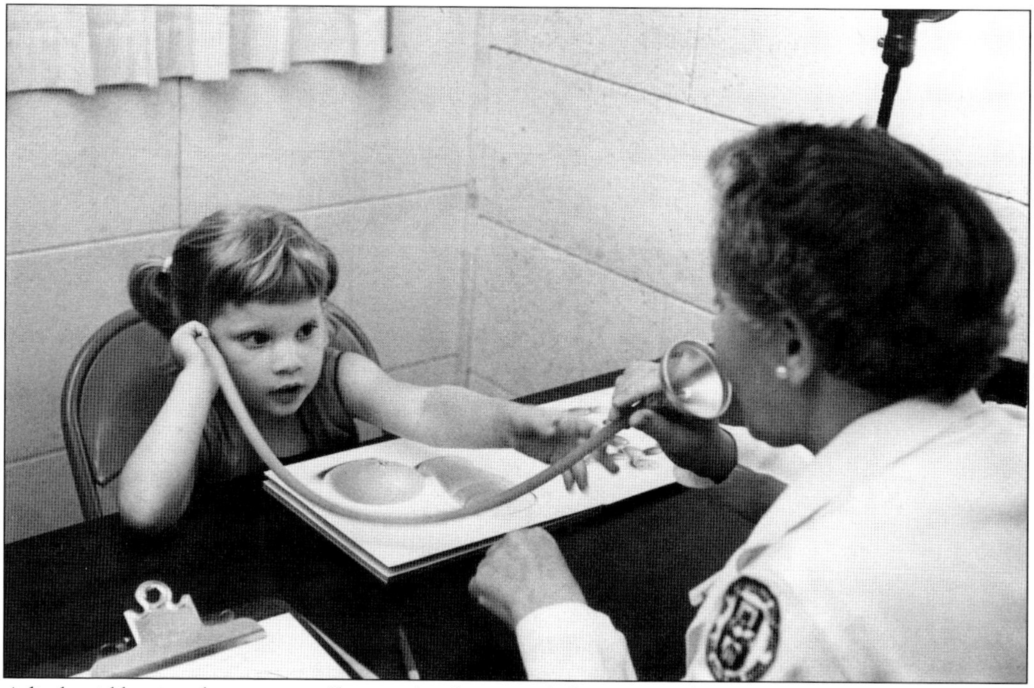

A little girl begins the process of having her hearing deficiency analyzed at the Lester N. Hofheimer Speech and Hearing Clinic in 1955. The *Stethoscope*, the medical center's monthly newsletter, reported that despite having some hearing loss, the patient "responded well to the training she received and now is able to go to nursery school." (Photograph by Werner Wolff.)

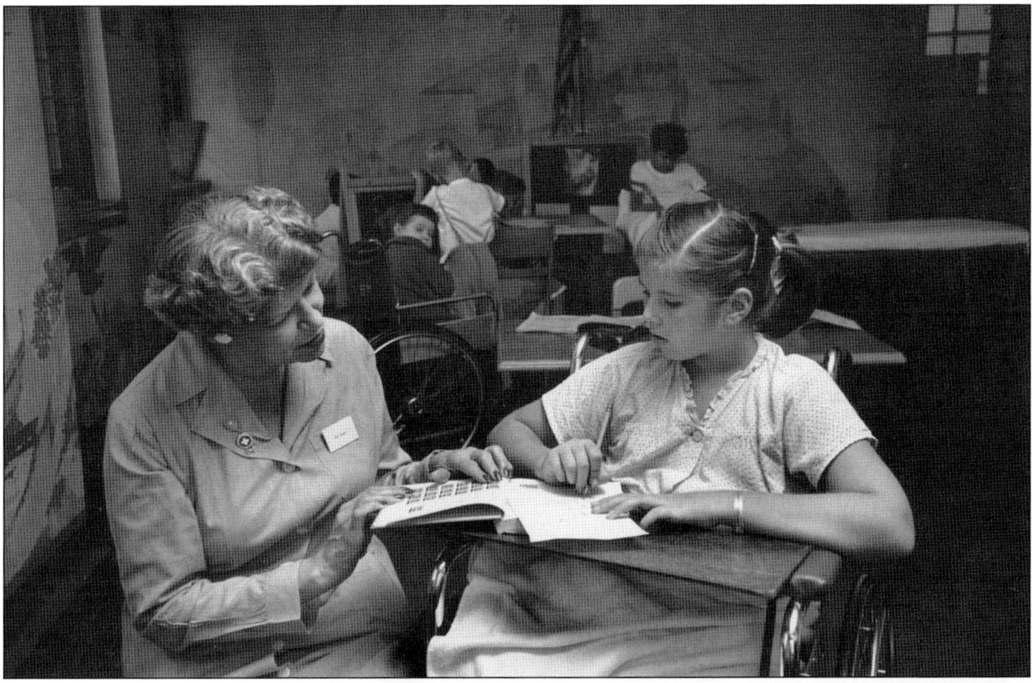

New York City Public School 401-X was a unique Babies Hospital feature for many years. Created for long-term hospital patients, the school enabled them to keep up with their schoolwork and helped them graduate on time. Though headed by a New York City public school teacher, much of the instruction was provided by hospital volunteers. The 1956 photograph above shows a volunteer assisting a patient in the schoolroom on the 12th floor of Babies Hospital. Occasionally, the school even had commencements; at right are two patients who were awarded their elementary school diplomas in a hospital rooftop ceremony in June 1951. (Above, photograph by Martin Iger; right, photograph by Lawrence G. Heinrich.)

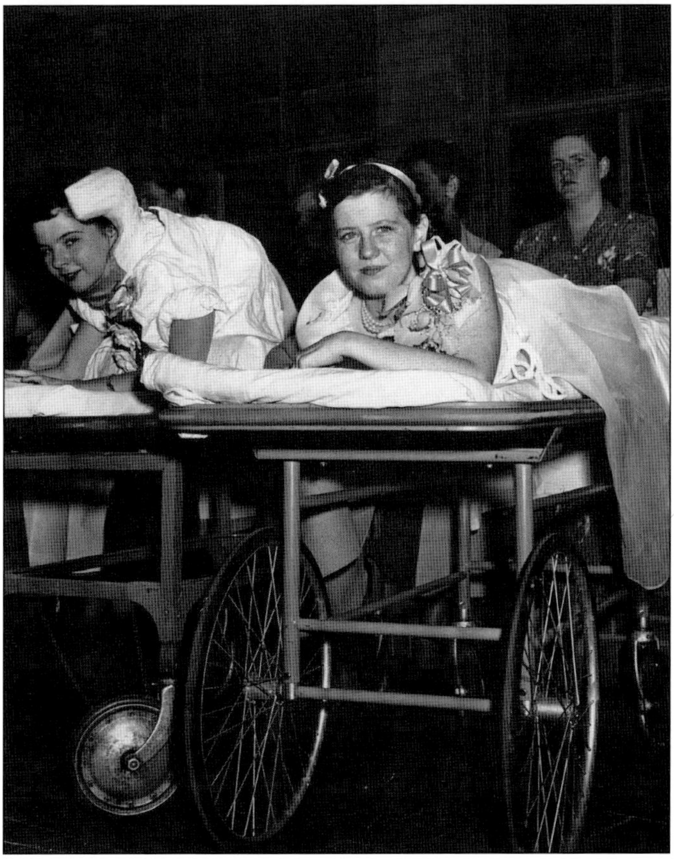

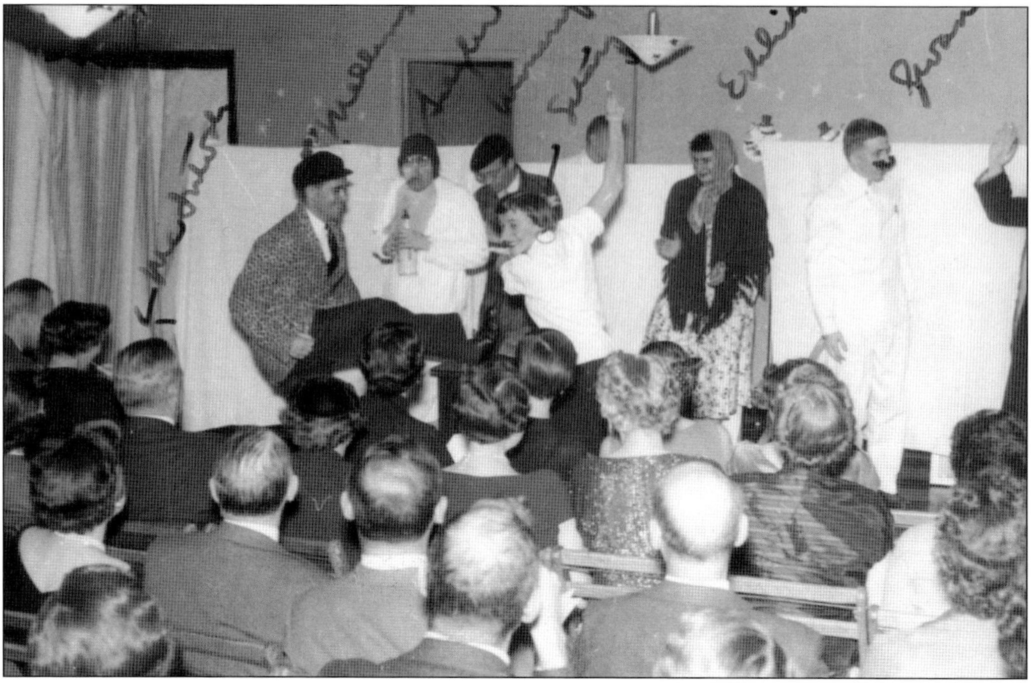

Faculty holiday parties, usually including comic skits performed by residents, have a long history at Babies Hospital. Identified onstage here during the 1956 party are, from left to right, Robert B. Mellins, Marvin M. Siegler, Robert W. Moncrieff, Anneliese L. Sitarz, Fred Erhlich, and Thurman B. Givan Jr. Babies Hospital director Rustin McIntosh is identified in the audience. Mellins became a leading authority on childhood asthma, while Sitarz was a pioneering pediatric oncologist.

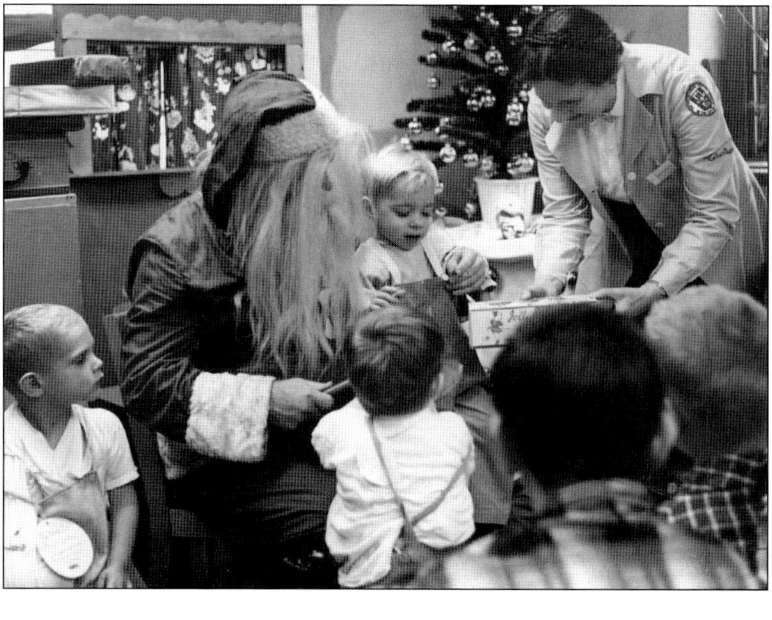

Children gather around Santa Claus for their gifts, which a volunteer helps distribute, while others wait expectantly. In 1957, Santa was Dr. John C. Dower, who was serving as an assistant resident. Dower would become president of the Babies Hospital Alumni Association in 1992. (Photograph by Elizabeth Wilcox.)

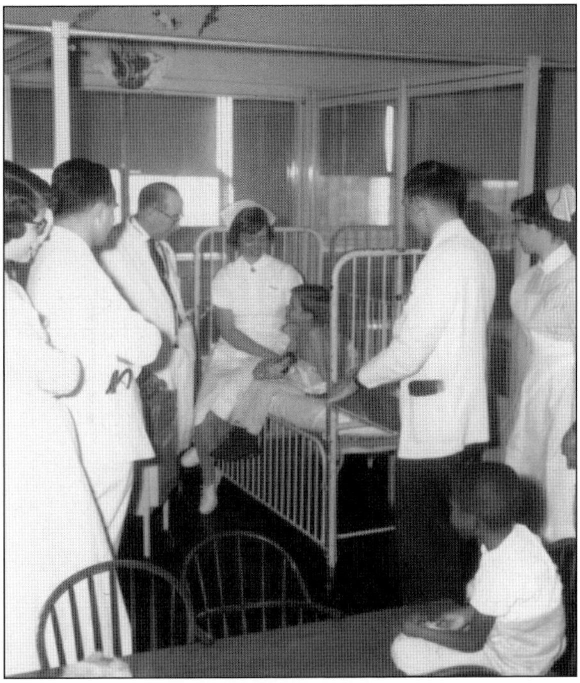

Babies Hospital pioneered the treatment and research of childhood nephrosis, a kidney disease characterized by, among other things, swelling of the tissues. Starting in the 1940s, Drs. Conrad Riley and Alice Davis established a nephrosis clinic and research program at the hospital. They treated patients with steroids such as ACTH (adrenocorticotropic hormone) and cortisone and reported reduced swelling and longer life expectancies in their patients. At left, a patient suffering from the disease is examined during ward rounds in Babies Hospital in 1958. The staff is unidentified. Below, a physician checks the eyes of another nephrosis patient. Besides his work on nephrosis, Riley also identified a rare genetic disorder that affected the nervous system now known as Riley-Day syndrome. (Both photographs by Elizabeth Wilcox.)

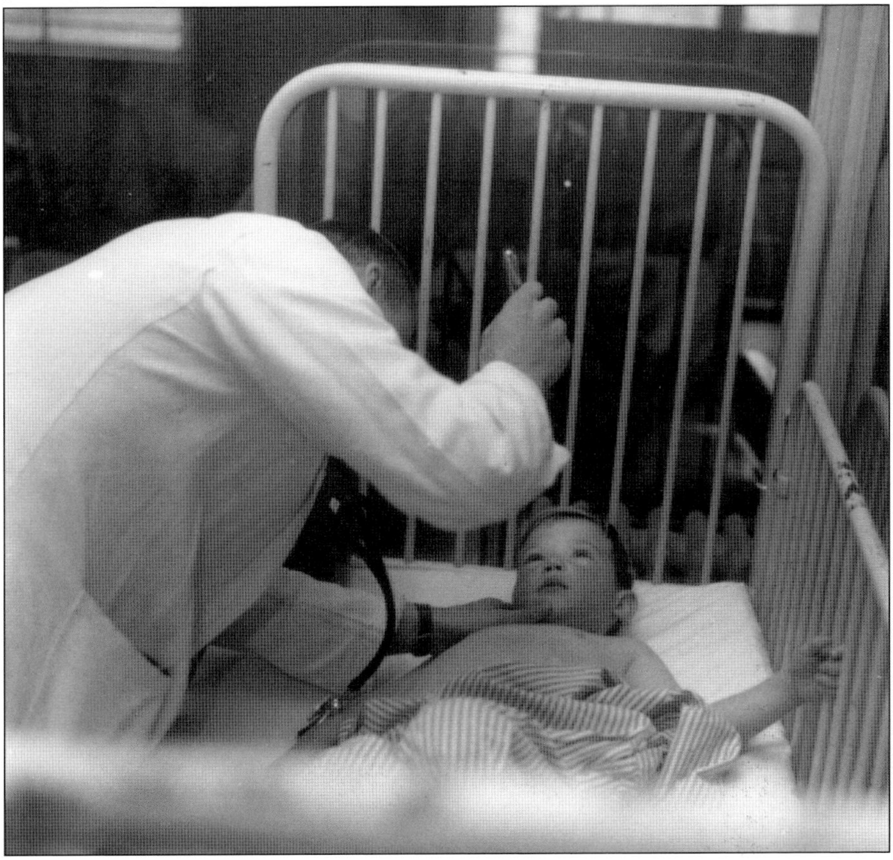

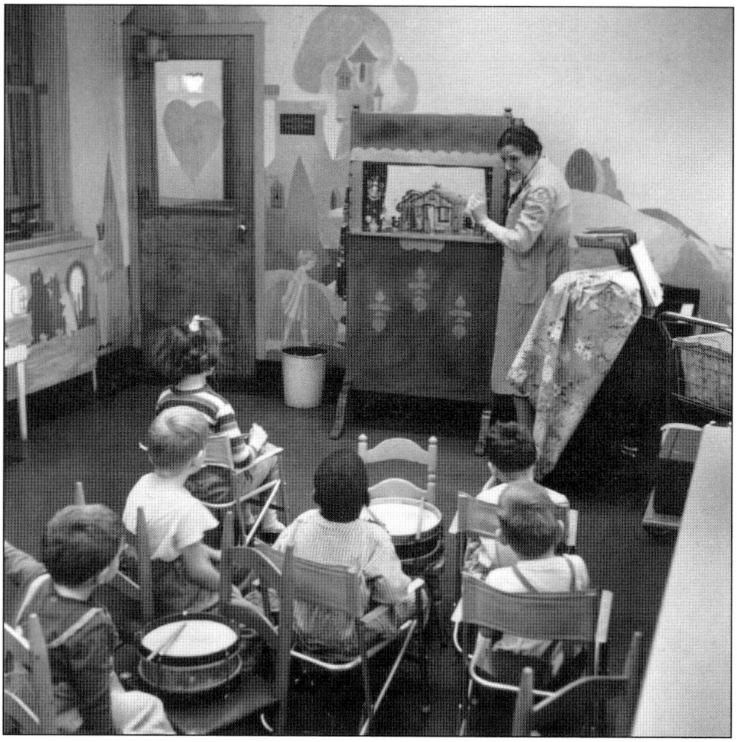

Patients are entertained with a puppet show in the playroom on the 12th floor of Babies Hospital in 1958. Well-equipped rooms for play and other activities for long-term patients have a lengthy history at Babies Hospital. The family of FAO Schwartz, owner of the famous toy store, provided the funds for building and equipping the first playrooms when Babies Hospital moved to the Columbia-Presbyterian Medical Center in 1929. (Photograph by Elizabeth Wilcox.)

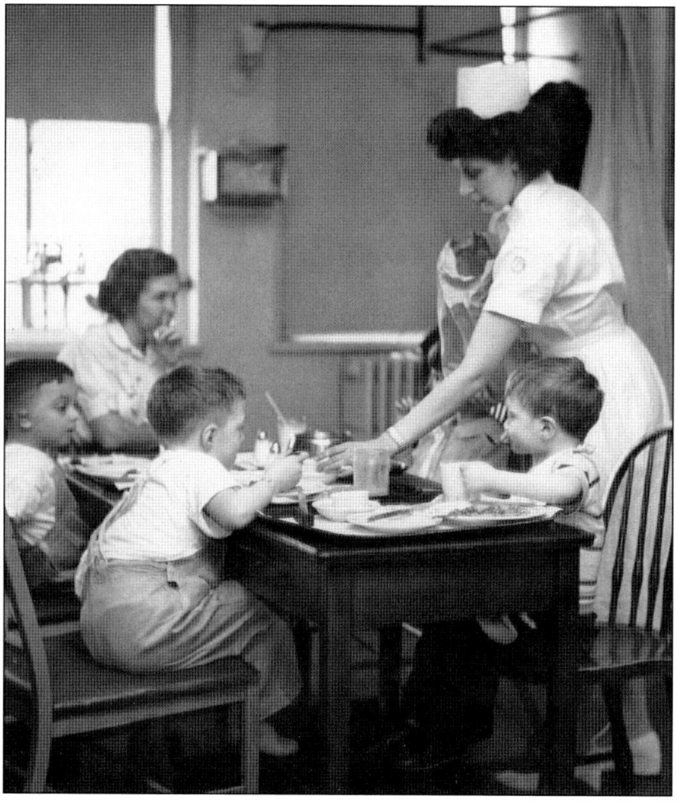

Children enjoy lunch at Babies Hospital in 1958. These were long-term patients, something much more common in the 1950s than today. A table of four was the norm and provided a home-like setting for the patients. The woman at right is probably a nurse's aide, while the one at left is most likely a volunteer. (Photograph by Elizabeth Wilcox.)

A student from the Presbyterian Hospital–Columbia University School of Nursing (now the Columbia University School of Nursing) weighs a patient at Babies Hospital in 1958. Nursing students were an important source of patient care at the hospital throughout its history. By the 1958–1959 academic year, School of Nursing students were required to take 90 hours of pediatric training at Babies Hospital. (Photograph by Elizabeth Wilcox.)

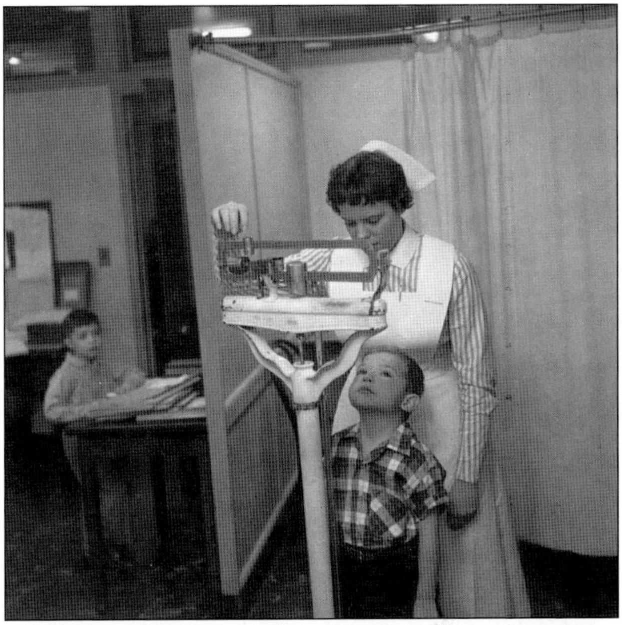

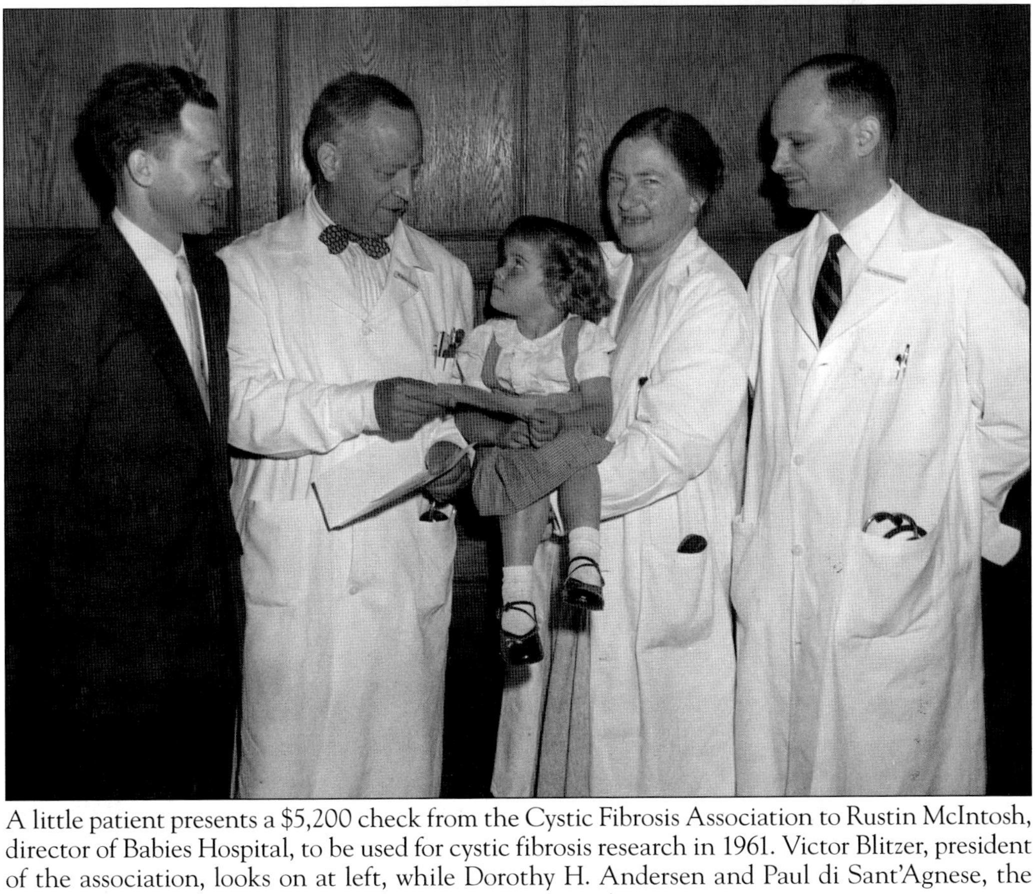

A little patient presents a $5,200 check from the Cystic Fibrosis Association to Rustin McIntosh, director of Babies Hospital, to be used for cystic fibrosis research in 1961. Victor Blitzer, president of the association, looks on at left, while Dorothy H. Andersen and Paul di Sant'Agnese, the physicians who would direct the research, are on the right.

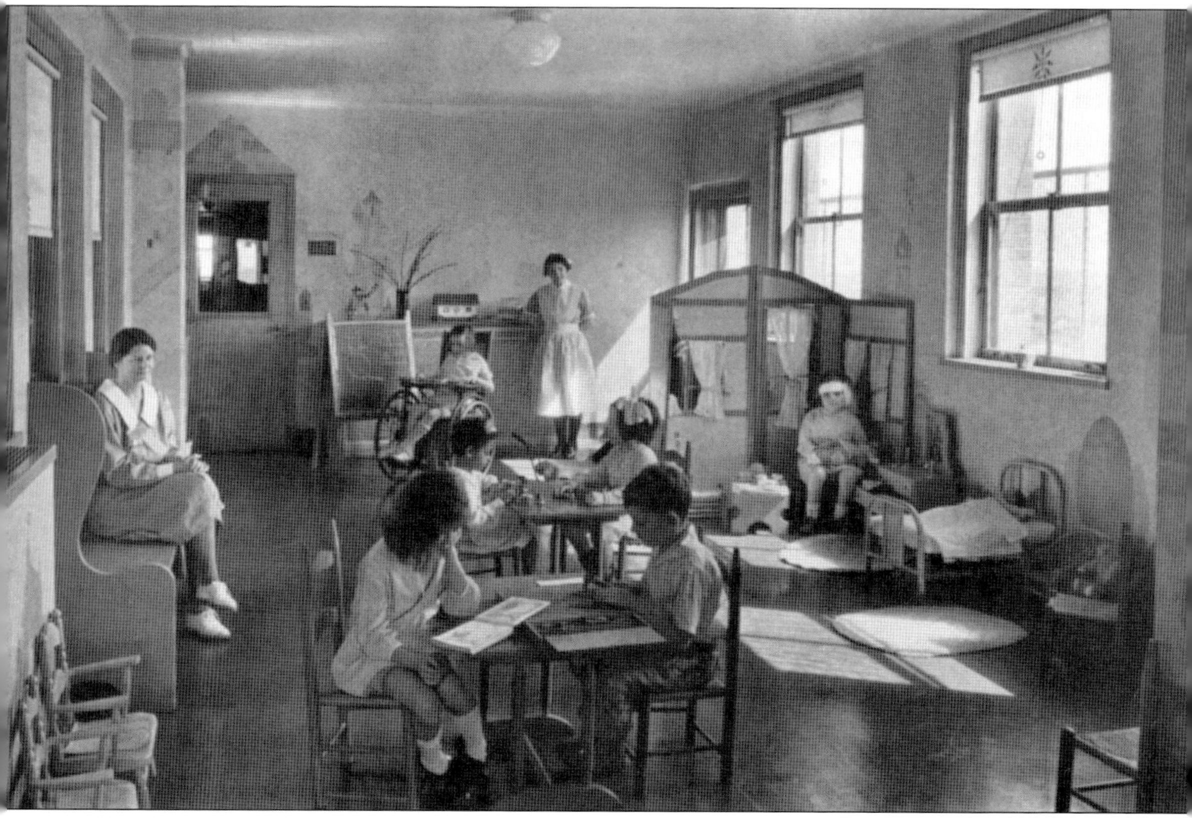

The Babies Hospital department of educational therapy classroom is seen here in an image from the 1931 annual report. While the department made sure its students remained caught up with their schoolwork, its philosophy was very much one of enhanced learning: "Geography is taught not alone from text book, but through map making, pictures, and stories." There was story hour two mornings a week, the report noted, "with more than thirty books selected from children's classics. . . . This has provided not only entertainment, but also a wider background in familiarity with fine literature, with the use of good grammar, enlarged vocabularies, and includes the hope of instilling the love of good reading for itself." Arts and crafts included "basketry, clay modeling, geometric design, sewing cards, knitting and crochet work, and paper construction in form of projects for Hallowe'en, Thanksgiving, Christmas, Valentine's Day, and Easter." The report noted that "thanks to the generous gift of a piano from Dr. McIntosh the children have enjoyed singing and have learned twenty songs including Christmas carols and folk melodies."

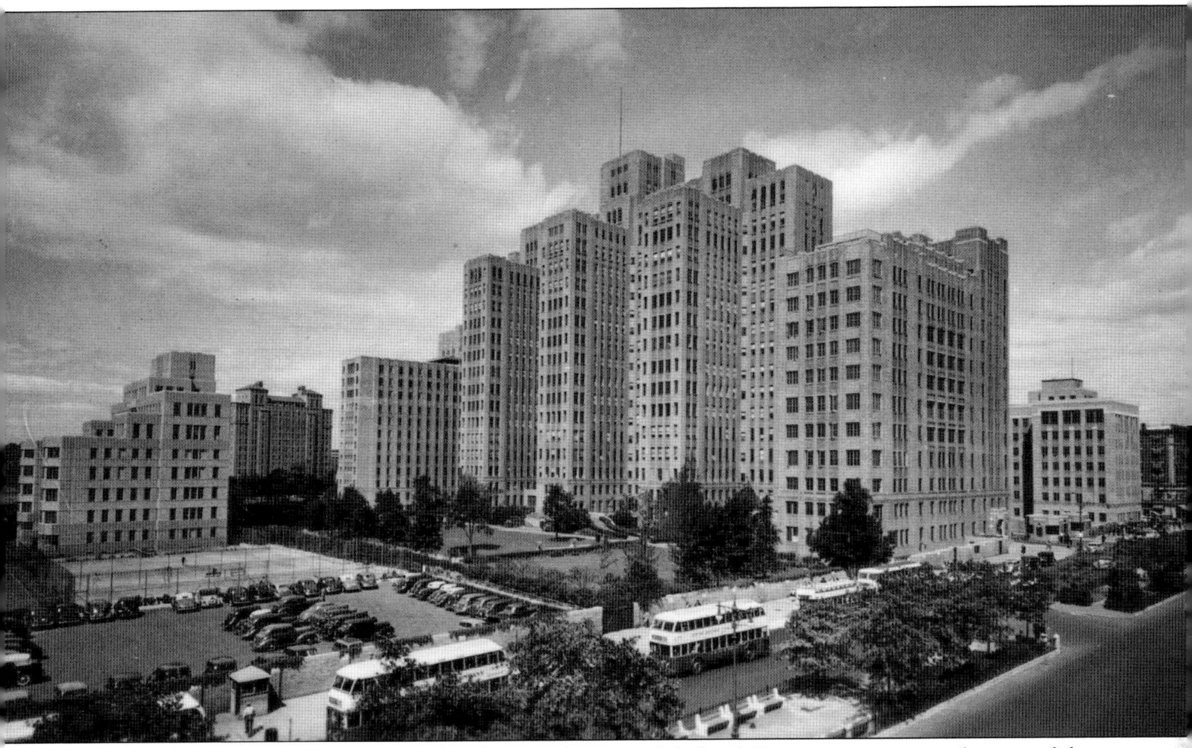

This c. 1945 postcard shows the Columbia-Presbyterian Medical Center as it was on the eve of the postwar era. Babies Hospital is seen at right center, facing Broadway. To its right is the Washington Heights Health Center at the corner of West 168th Street, constructed in 1938–1939 by the New York City Department of Health. To the left, the Babies Hospital overlooks part of the medical center garden (now the site of the hospital's Central Building) and beyond that a parking lot at the corner of Broadway and West 165th Street, which, almost 60 years later, would become the location of the Morgan Stanley Children's Hospital. The rest of the campus seen here is, from left to right, the Harkness Institute of Ophthalmology, the School of Nursing's Anna Maxwell Hall (razed in 1983–1984 to make way for the Milstein Hospital Building), the Harkness Pavilion, and the main complex housing Presbyterian Hospital and the College of Physicians and Surgeons. Broadway's spacious center medians and its double-decker buses are both unfortunately things of the past.

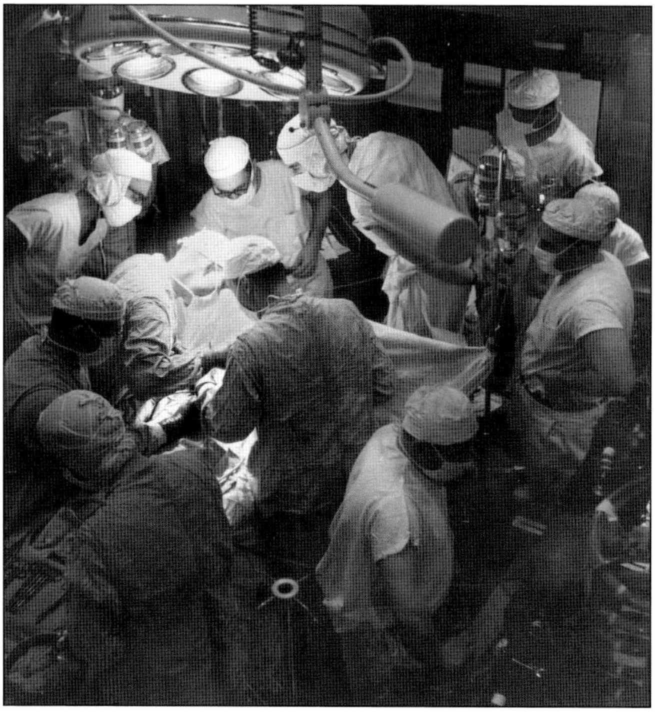

Pediatric open-heart surgery is seen in progress in 1958 at left. Open-heart surgery of any kind was still cutting-edge then, let alone those involving children, and the persons on the fringes of this group were not participating in the operation but rather surgeons observing a novel procedure. Dr. James Malm is said to have been the lead surgeon for this operation, though he is not identified in the image. Malm would go on to become one of the country's leading pediatric heart surgeons. In the 1974 photograph below, he is shown with twin sisters, age four, whom he had successfully operated on for a heart condition. (Left, photograph by Elizabeth Wilcox; below, photograph by Lucy Lazzopina.)

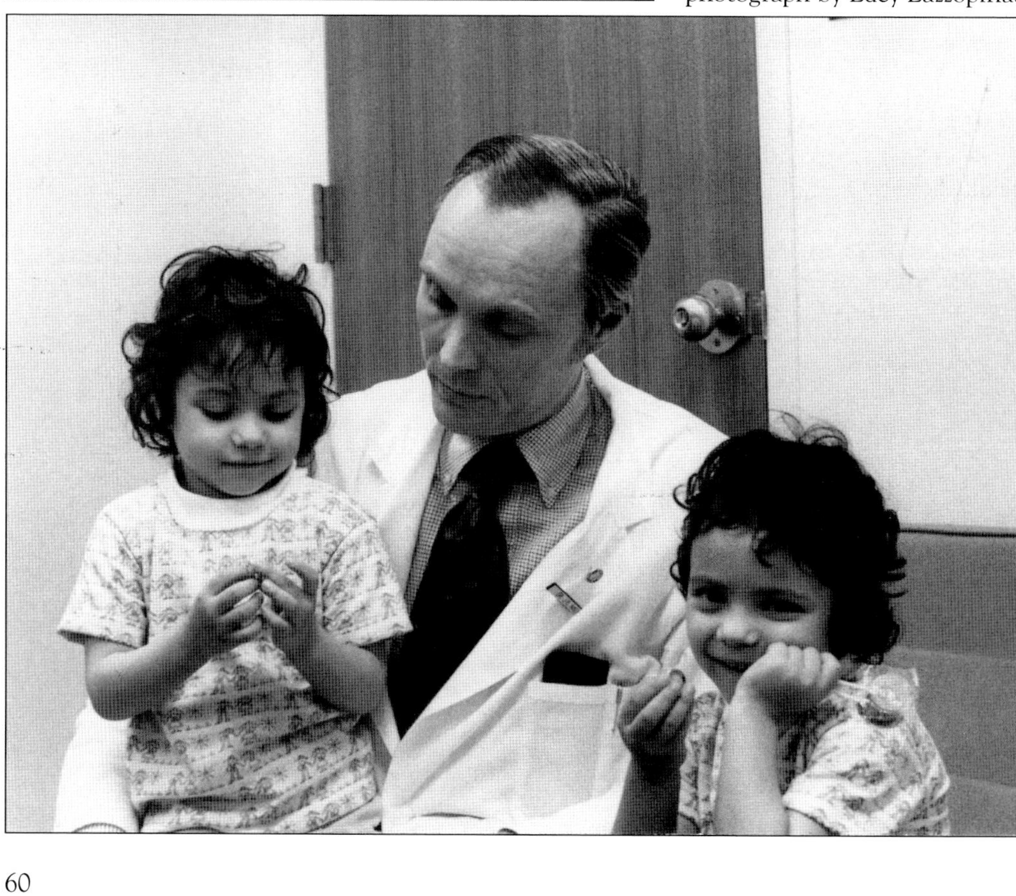

Four

The Birth of Pediatric Subspecialties

The 30-year tenure of Rustin McIntosh, MD, as the Carpentier Professor of Pediatrics at the College of Physicians & Surgeon of Columbia University and the pediatrician-in-chief of the Babies Hospital witnessed the birth of six child-focused subspecialties that were among the very first in the United States.

Bernard Sachs, MD, one of the founders of the Neurological Institute at Columbia, the first specialty hospital in the United States devoted entirely to disorders of the nervous system, was the first director of child neurology. Sachs, collaborating with the English ophthalmologist Warren Tay, described the neurological aspects of Tay-Sachs disease.

Dr. Hattie Alexander, director of infectious disease, joined the faculty in 1932. She identified and studied antibiotic resistance and developed an antiserum that was the first effective treatment for *Haemophilus influenza*.

In 1938, Dorothy Andersen, jointly appointed in pediatrics and pathology, discovered and named cystic fibrosis (CF), a genetic disorder that affects the lungs, pancreas, and other organs, leading to life-threatening breathing and digestive problems.

As chief of the division of anesthesia in pediatrics, Virginia Apgar, MD, was the first woman to head a specialty division and to become a full tenured professor at the College of Physicians and Surgeons. Apgar developed a standardized scoring system to assess infant health at one minute and five minutes after birth. The Apgar score continues to be used in the 21st century to provide a convenient method for reporting the status of the newborn infant immediately after birth.

The division of newborn care evolved from the first unit dedicated to premature infants in the nation, created by Richard Lawrence Day, MD, at the Babies Hospital in 1949. William Silverman, a trainee of Dr. Day, became the first director of neonatology in the early 1950s and was regarded as the premier neonatologist of that period.

John Caffey is considered the father and innovator of the field of pediatric radiology. Dr. McIntosh, working with Ross Golden, MD, chair of radiology at Columbia-Presbyterian, created the first independent department of pediatric radiology in the early 1930s.

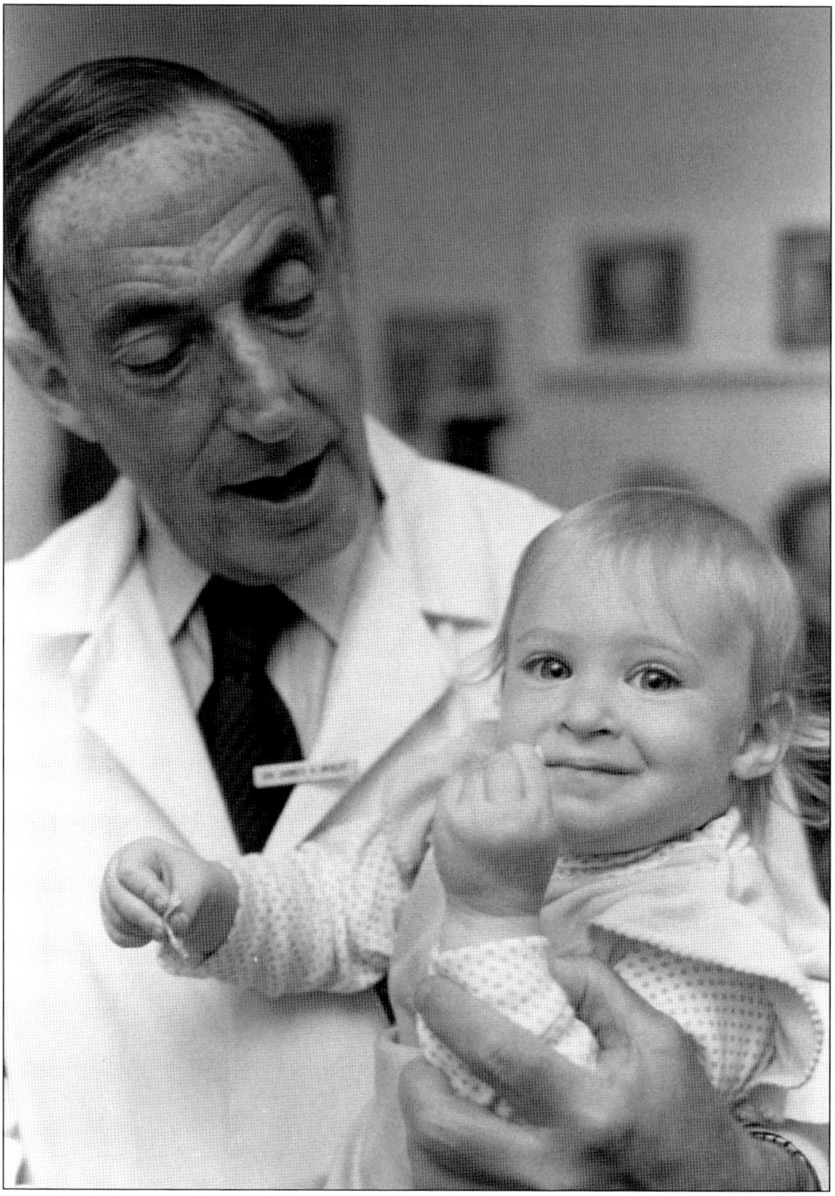

Dr. James Alexander Wolff, a pioneer in the field of pediatric hematology-oncology, was a native New Yorker who attended the Horace Mann School, graduated from Harvard University, and received his medical degree from New York University. Working with Drs. Louis Diamond and Sidney Farber at Boston Children's Hospital, he participated in one of the most important discoveries in pediatric medicine of the 20th century: the administration of Aminopterin to a child with leukemia. Their results, published in the *New England Journal of Medicine* in 1948, reported for the first time a complete remission in what had been a universally lethal disease. In 1959, Dr. Wolff was appointed the first full-time director of pediatric hematology-oncology at the Babies Hospital and Columbia's College of Physicians and Surgeons. He was a founding member of the Children's Leukemia Group B, which became the Children's Cancer Study Group. In 1996, he received the Distinguished Alumnus Award from Babies Hospital for his outstanding service, contributions to research, and mentorship to a generation of pediatric hematologists-oncologists.

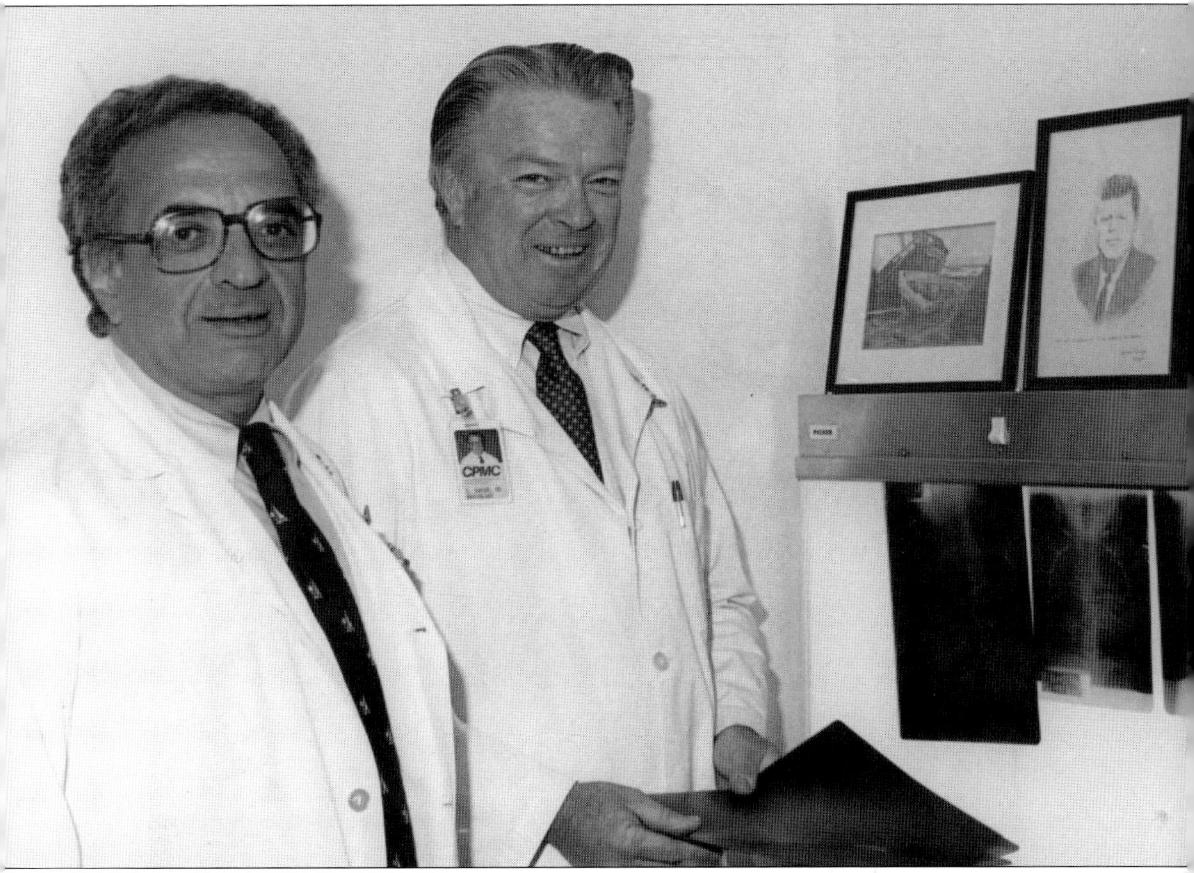

Dr. David H. Baker, at right, was uniquely trained in his field by the two fathers of pediatric radiology: Dr. John Caffey at Babies Hospital and Dr. Edward Newhauser at Boston Children's Hospital. Born in Concord, New Hampshire, in 1925, Dr. Baker served in Patton's Third Army and was wounded in the Battle of the Bulge. He attended Wesleyan University and received his medical doctorate from Boston University. He completed residencies in pediatrics and radiology at New York Hospital–Cornell Medical Center and joined the faculty at Babies Hospital in 1959, succeeding Dr. John Caffey as director of pediatric radiology. With his colleague Dr. Walter Berdon (left), he edited many editions of *Caffey's Textbook of Pediatric Radiology*. He and Dr. Berdon also published many early seminal articles on pediatric radiology and were responsible for describing the radiologic findings of both common and esoteric diseases of childhood. (Photograph by Arthur Pease.)

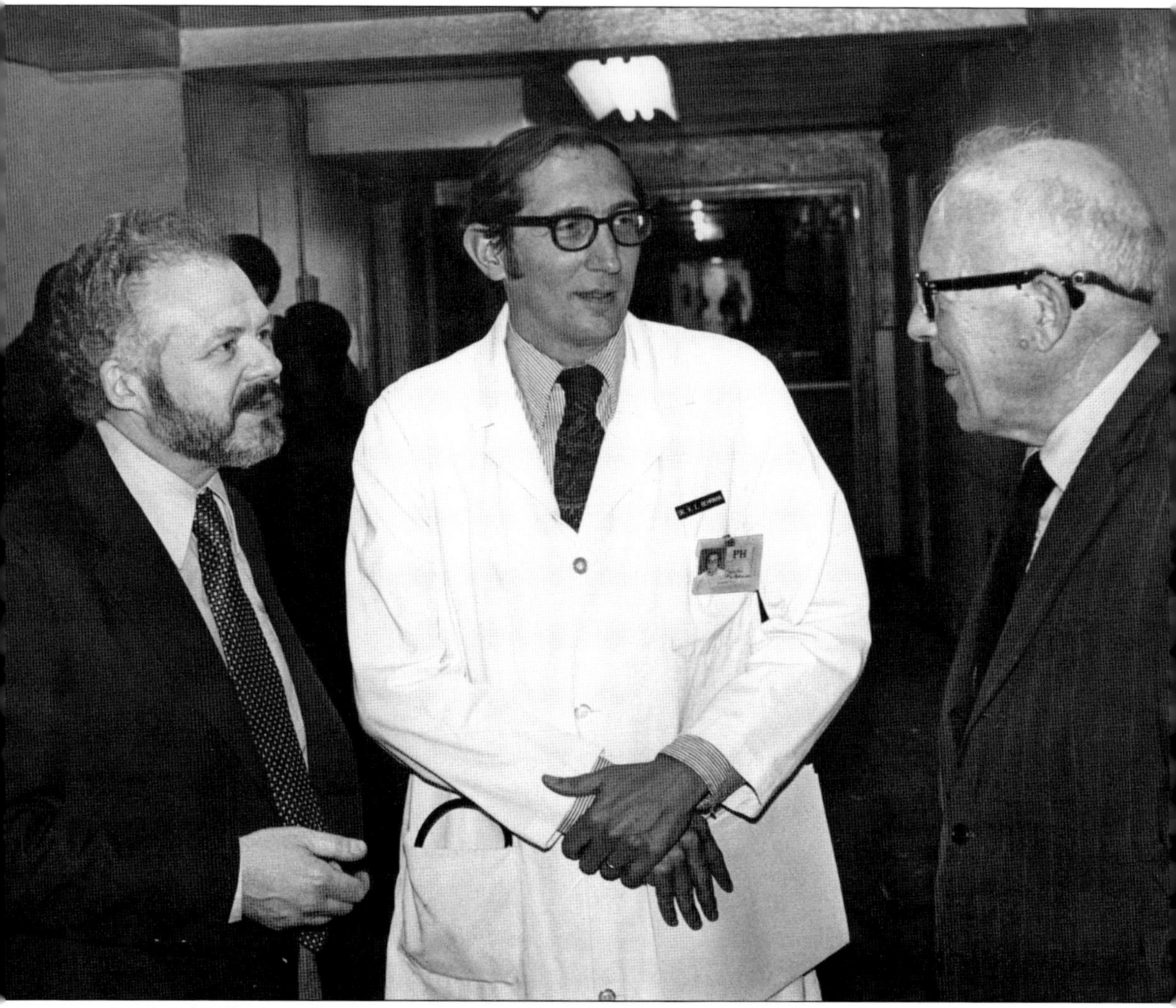

Richard Behrman (center) was born in Philadelphia and received an undergraduate degree from Amherst College, a juris doctor degree from Harvard, and a medical degree from the University of Rochester. He completed his pediatric residency at the Harriet Lane Service, Johns Hopkins University Hospital. Behrman was appointed the Reuben S. Carpentier Professor and chair of the Department of Pediatrics at the Babies Hospital, Columbia-Presbyterian Medical Center, in 1971, a position he occupied until 1976. Behrman left Columbia to serve as chair of pediatrics and dean at Case Western Reserve School of Medicine. In 1989, Stanford University recruited him to plan its new Lucille Packard Children's Hospital, which opened in 1991. Simultaneously, he led important initiatives at the David and Lucille Packard Foundation, particularly its Center for the Future of Children, an interdisciplinary team that conducted research and grant-making on children's issues. Dr. Behrman later became senior health advisor at the foundation. He passed away in 2020.

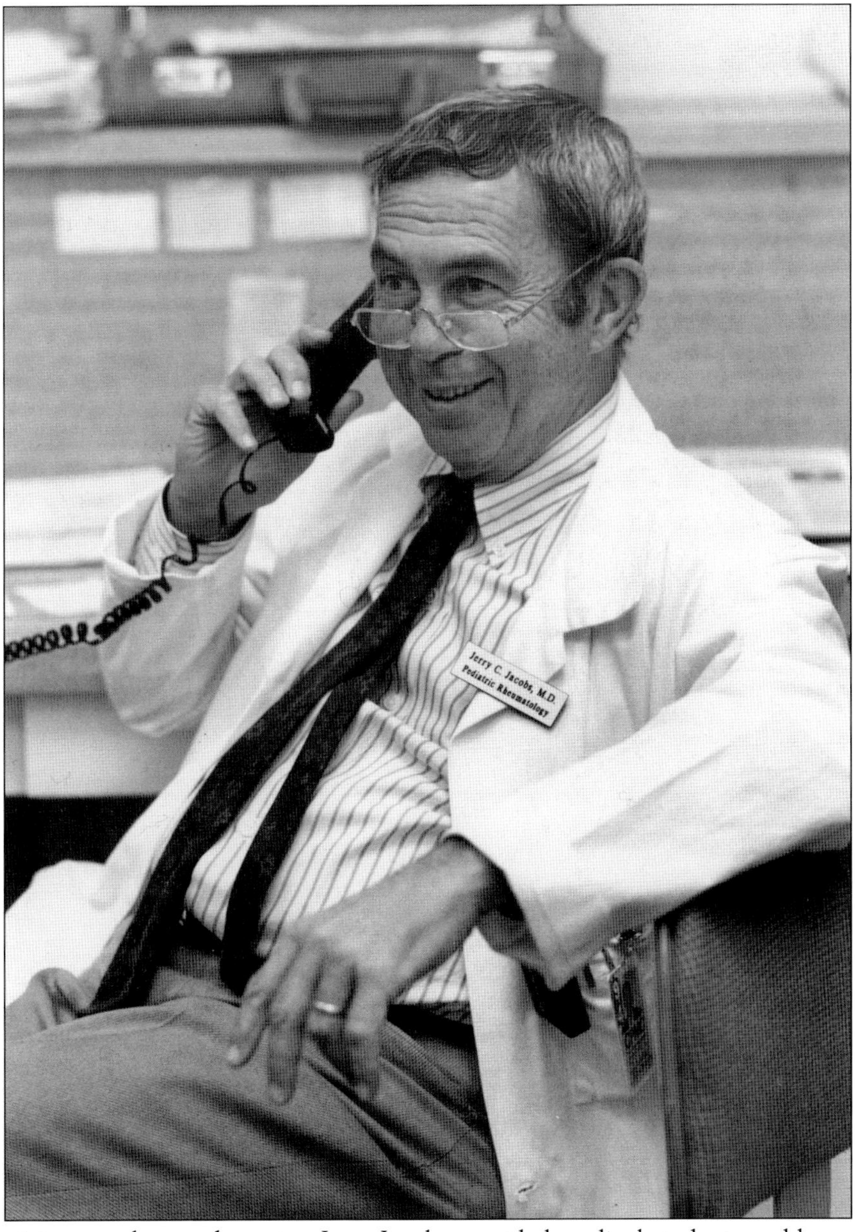

A pediatrician, teacher, and mentor, Jerry Jacobs provided medical students and house staff at Babies Hospital and Columbia University with an indelible model of the responsible physician. In 1960, he founded the division of pediatric rheumatology at the Babies Hospital and was pediatrician-in-chief at the Edward Daniels Faulkner Arthritis Clinic of the Columbia-Presbyterian Medical Center. He was instrumental in creating the Regional Arthritis Program for Children (RAP4-KIDS) at the medical center, which provided community education and outreach, patient education and support services, and coordination of clinical and clinic support services. He pioneered the concept of the rapid mobilization of the child with arthritis and refused to allow chronic disease to interfere with his patients' normal childhood activities. In 1997, Dr. Jacobs was named a Master by the American Rheumatology Association. He was the author of a textbook, *Pediatric Rheumatology for the Practitioner.*

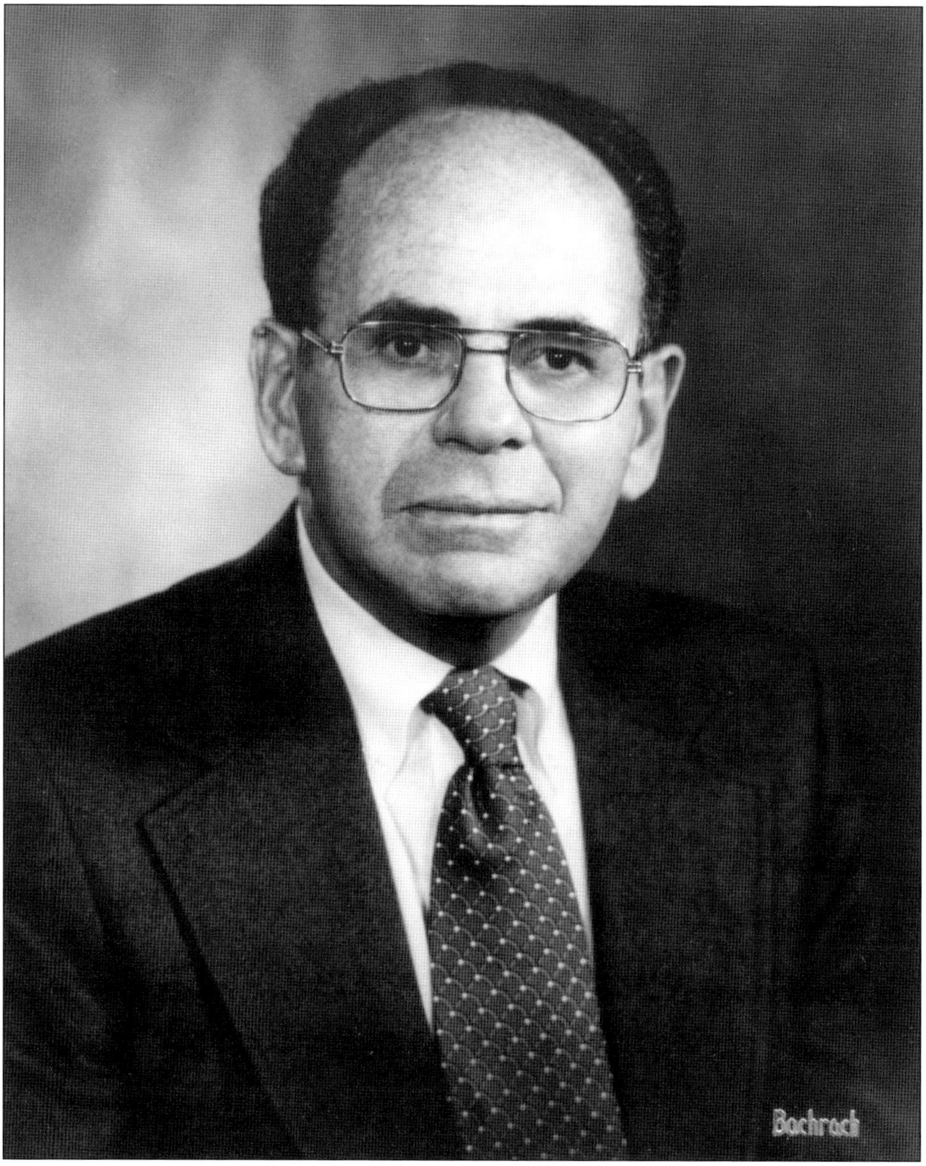

Born in Boston and educated at Dartmouth College and Boston University School of Medicine, Sidney Carter trained with Dr. H. Houston Merritt first at the Harvard Unit of Boston City Hospital and subsequently at Columbia. One day in 1951, Dr. Merritt phoned him and said, "Sid, I want you to head pediatric neurology." When Dr. Carter protested that he did not know much about pediatrics, Merritt, always pithy and laconic, replied with one word: "learn." Carter served as chief of child neurology until 1978 and is recognized as a founding member of child neurology as a recognized subspecialty in the United States. Dr. Carter built on this progress by establishing training and certification guidelines. In 1965, he received the first National Institutes of Health pediatric neurology training grant. He was instrumental in the 1968 decision by the American Board of Psychiatry and Neurology to grant certification in pediatric neurology. He is credited with making Columbia the center of child neurology in the United States for more than 25 years. He served as president of both the American Academy of Neurology and the American Neurological Association.

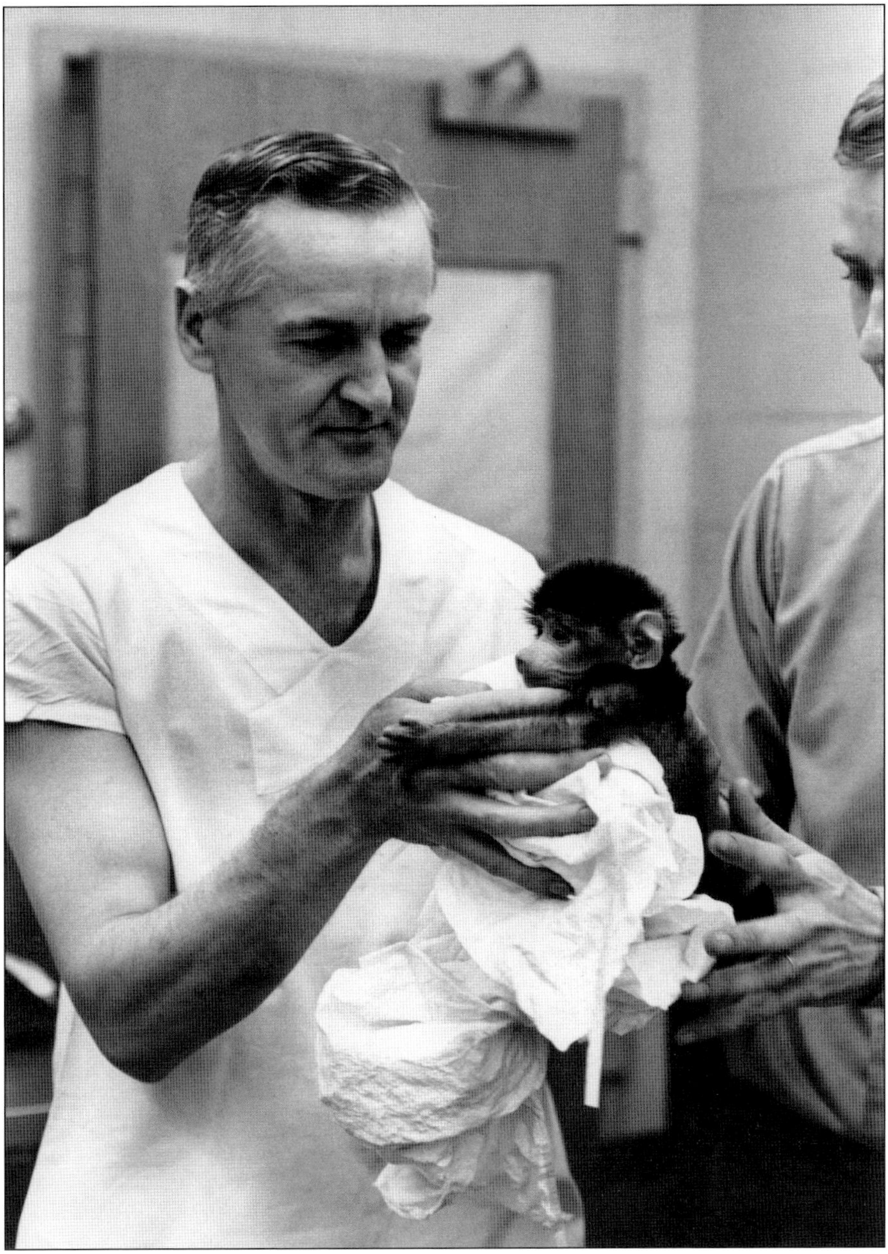

Dr. L. Stanley James earned a medical degree in his native New Zealand and joined the faculty of pediatrics and of obstetrics-gynecology at the Columbia University College of Physicians and Surgeons in 1959. He served as the director of perinatal medicine at the Babies Hospital for two decades beginning in 1972. Dr. James was one of the fathers of modern neonatal care. He joined Virginia Apgar to establish the scientific basis for the Apgar score and to identify key factors that adversely influence the health of newborns. His findings led to improvements in the care of newborns through resuscitation and the management of asphyxiation. James received the E. Mead Johnson Award and the Virginia Apgar Award from the American Academy of Pediatrics (AAP) and the Ronald McDonald Children's Charities Award for his contributions to the care of the fetus and newborn infants. (Photograph by Elizabeth Wilcox.)

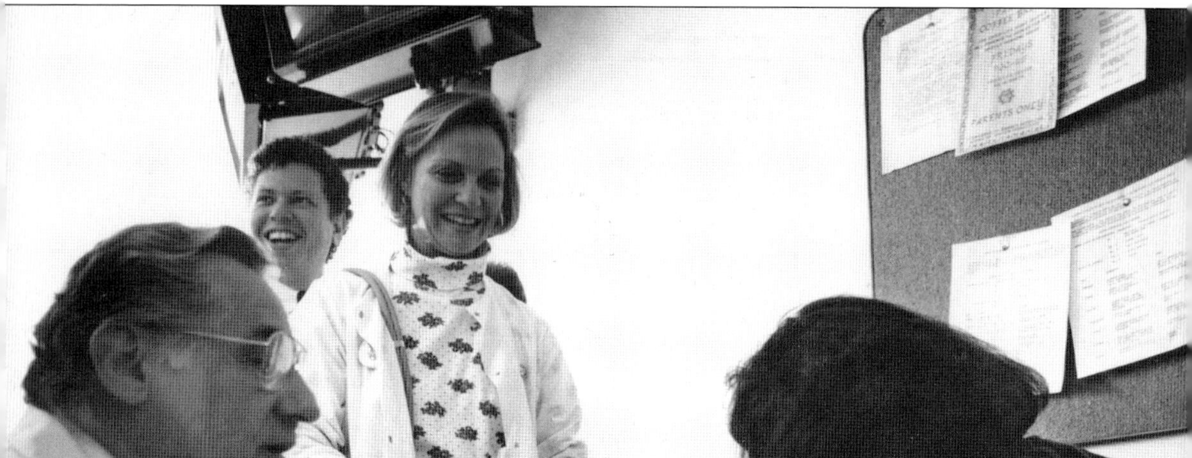

Darryl C. De Vivo, MD, received his medical degree from the University of Virginia and completed his pediatric and neurology residencies at Harvard, the National Institutes of Health, and Washington University. He joined the Columbia faculty in 1979 as the Sidney Carter Professor of Neurology, professor of pediatrics, and director of the pediatric neurology service. Currently, he continues to fulfill his duties as founding director of the Colleen Giblin Research Laboratories; director of the Pediatric Neuromuscular Disease Center; codirector of the Center for Motor Neuron Biology and Diseases (MNC); and associate chairman (neurology) for pediatric neurosciences. Dr. De Vivo was a director for neurology and president of the American Board of Psychiatry and Neurology, secretary of the American Academy of Neurology, and president of the Child Neurology Society. He has published more than 450 original articles and reviews and is a former associate editor for the textbook *Rudolph's Pediatrics*. He is a current editor of *Neuromuscular Disorders in Infancy, Childhood and Adolescence: A Clinician's Approach*.

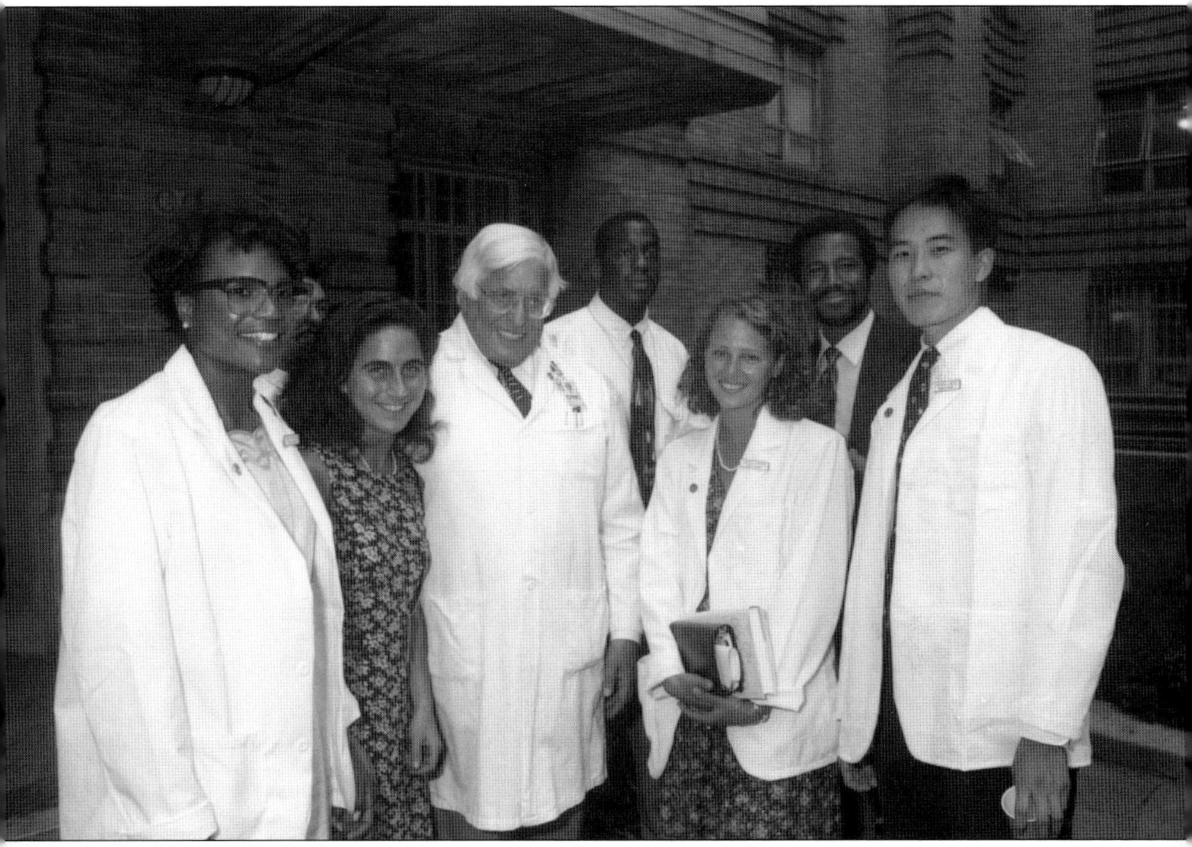

Dr. Arnold Gold (center), a renowned pediatric neurologist and master diagnostician, became an international advocate for humanism in health care. A pioneer in child neurology, he treated thousands of children and provided a model of skill, knowledge, and compassion for the countless pediatric residents and medical students who trained with him. Dr. Lewis P. Rowland, former chair of neurology at Columbia University, said of Dr. Gold, "Arnold's patients come before all else. He is legendary in his ability to calm the most anxious . . . distressed child. Residents and medical students flock to him—not just because he is so stimulating but because he serves as such a role model." Dr. Gold and his wife, Sandra, cofounded the Arnold P. Gold Foundation with an aim toward sustaining the human connection in medicine and ensuring all patients received compassionate care. The Arnold P. Gold Foundation's programs, such as the White Coat Ceremony and the Gold Humanism Honor Society, are now found in nearly every medical school in the country and many schools throughout the world to promote compassion and humanism in future doctors.

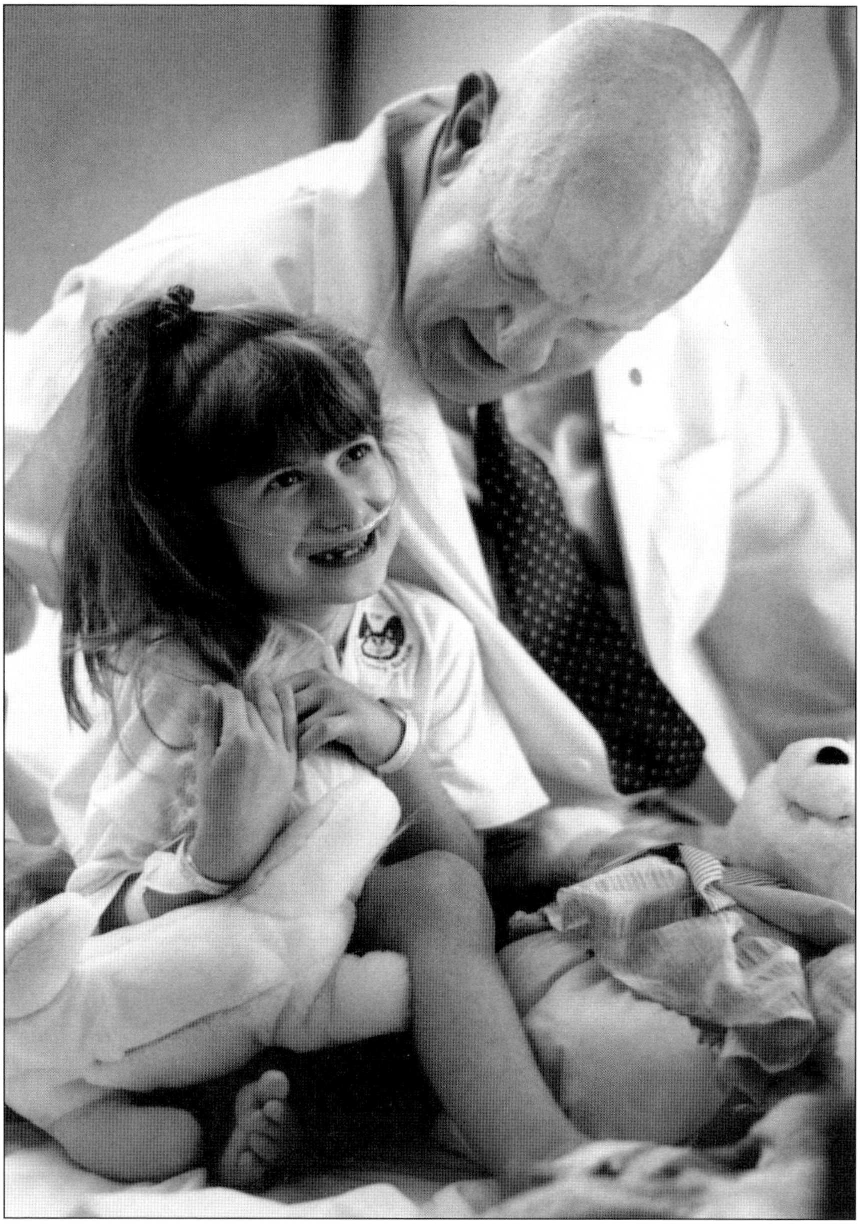

John Driscoll attended Hamilton College, where he was cocaptain of the varsity basketball and lacrosse teams as well as president of the graduating class of 1958. He completed medical school at Wake Forest University, served in the Navy, completed a pediatric residency at Babies Hospital, and joined the faculty in 1971. Driscoll was named the director of the neonatal intensive care unit and division chief of neonatology. In 1997, he was appointed the Reuben S. Carpentier Professor and chair of the department of pediatrics at Columbia University College of Physicians and Surgeons and physician-in-chief, Babies Hospital, Columbia-Presbyterian Medical Center. During his tenure, new divisions of emergency medicine, critical care, and molecular genetics were created. In 1998, Columbia-Presbyterian merged with the New York Hospital to become the NewYork-Presbyterian Hospital (NYPH), and a new children's hospital, the Morgan Stanley Children's Hospital, was born in 2003. The name Babies Hospital of New York, therefore, no longer existed.

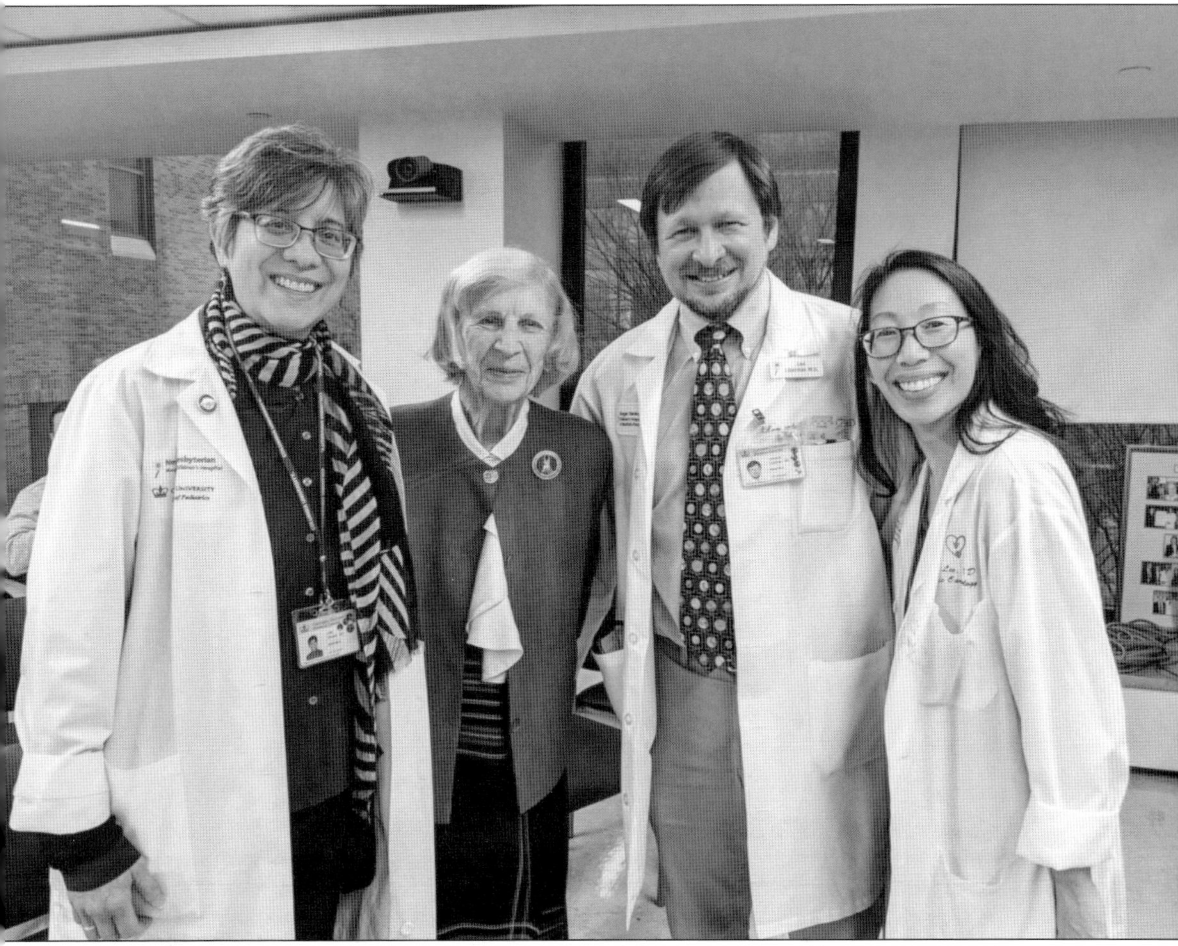

Sylvia Griffiths, a New York City native, graduated from Hunter College in 1944 and earned her medical degree from the Yale University School of Medicine in 1948. In 1955, she came to Columbia and with Dr. Sidney Blumenthal established the division of pediatric cardiology at the Babies Hospital, Columbia Presbyterian Medical Center. Dr. Griffiths is recognized as a pioneer in pediatric cardiology as well as a consummate clinician, esteemed teacher, and mentor. In 1960, she was named one of the 50 founders of the Subspecialty Board of Pediatric Cardiology. At Columbia, she directed the Pediatric Cardiac Clinic from 1972 to 1990, becoming professor of clinical pediatrics in 1977. She is the author of more than 150 scientific publications. In 1996, her colleagues and former students established the Sylvia P. Griffiths, MD, Lectureship and Teaching Day, held annually to honor her outstanding humanistic qualities and her dedication to teaching. Pictured in this photograph from the December 13, 2018, lecture are, from left to right, Julie Vincent, MD, director of pediatric cardiology; Dr. Griffiths; Leo Liberman, MD; and Teresa Lee, MD.

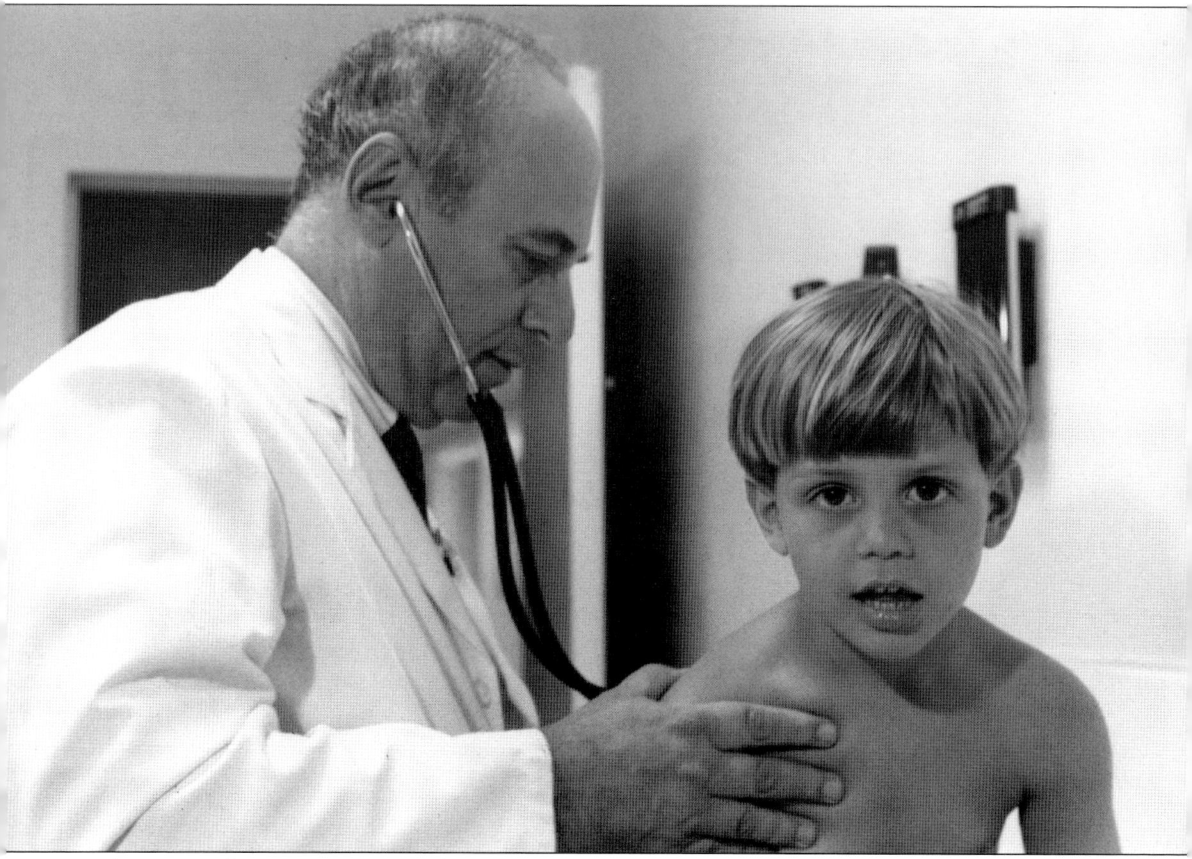

A native of Syracuse, New York, Welton Gersony received his medical degree from the State University of New York–Upstate Medical Center in 1958. He completed a pediatric residency at Cleveland Children's Hospital and, after serving in the US Army Medical Corps, completed his pediatric cardiology training at Boston Children's Hospital, Harvard Medical School. He joined the faculty at the Columbia-Presbyterian Medical Center's Babies Hospital in 1968 as the Alexander Nadas Professor of Pediatrics. He was also director of the division of pediatric cardiology at the hospital, a position he served in for 35 years. Dr. Gersony's area of expertise is the natural history of congenital heart disease, and he was the principal investigator on the collaborative studies on the natural history of congenital heart defects and the author of the textbook *Congenital Heart Disease in the Adult*. He received the American Heart Association's Distinguished Service Award and the Founders Award of the American Academy of Pediatrics.

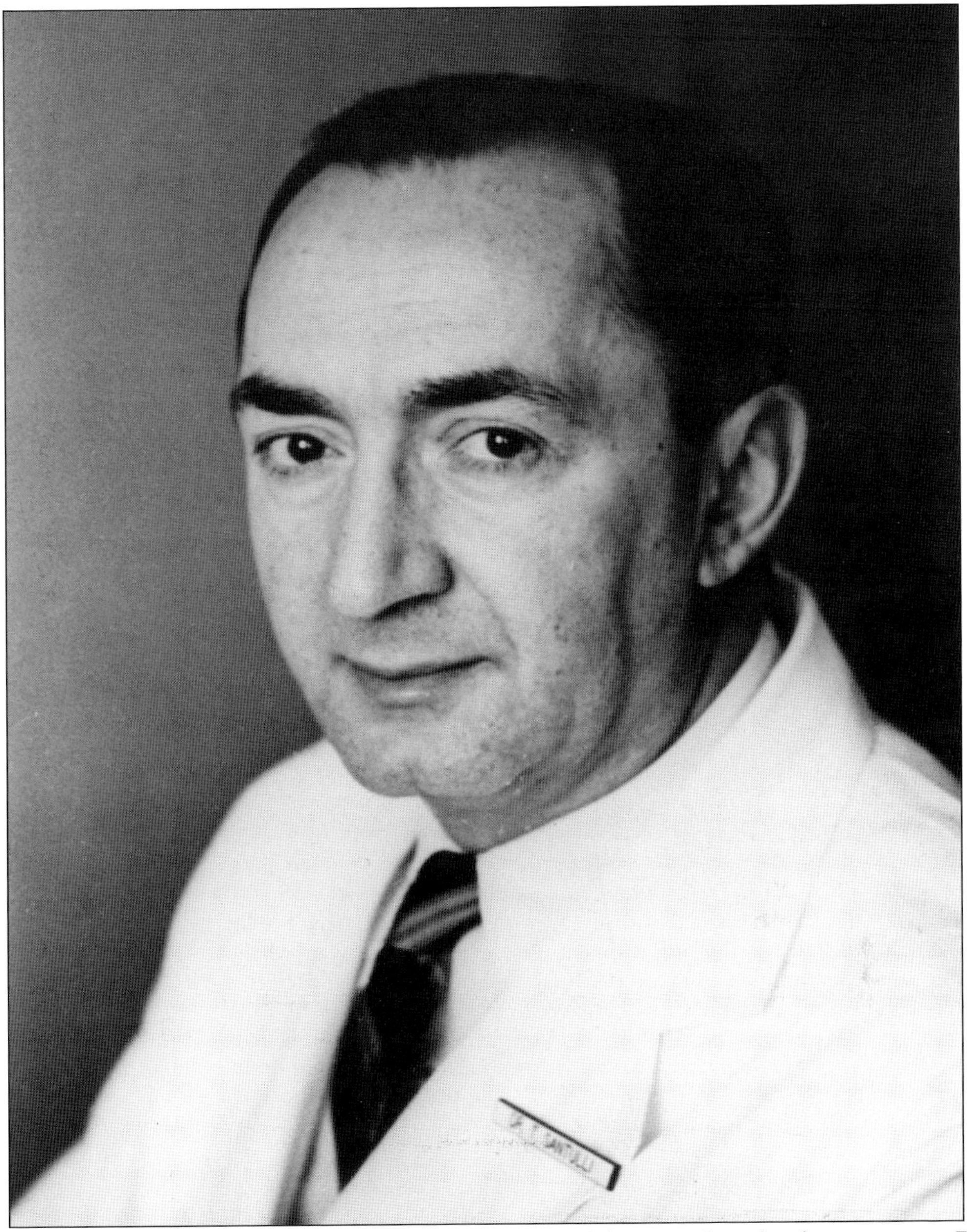

Thomas V. Santulli was a pioneer in the development of the specialty of pediatric surgery. Dr. Santulli received a bachelor of science degree from Columbia University in 1935 and his medical degree from Georgetown University in 1939. He joined the faculty of the Babies Hospital and remained on staff for his more-than-40-year professional career. Dr. Santulli was president of the American Pediatric Surgical Association, the first president of the New York Pediatric Surgical Society, and a member of the American Surgical Association, the New York Surgical Society, the British Association of Pediatric Surgeons, and the American College of Surgeons. When he retired as an emeritus professor in 1983, the pediatric surgery library and conference room at Babies Hospital were named in his honor. He received Babies Hospital's Centennial Medal as the "Father of Pediatric Surgery." His legacy also is reflected in the Santulli lectureship in pediatric surgery.

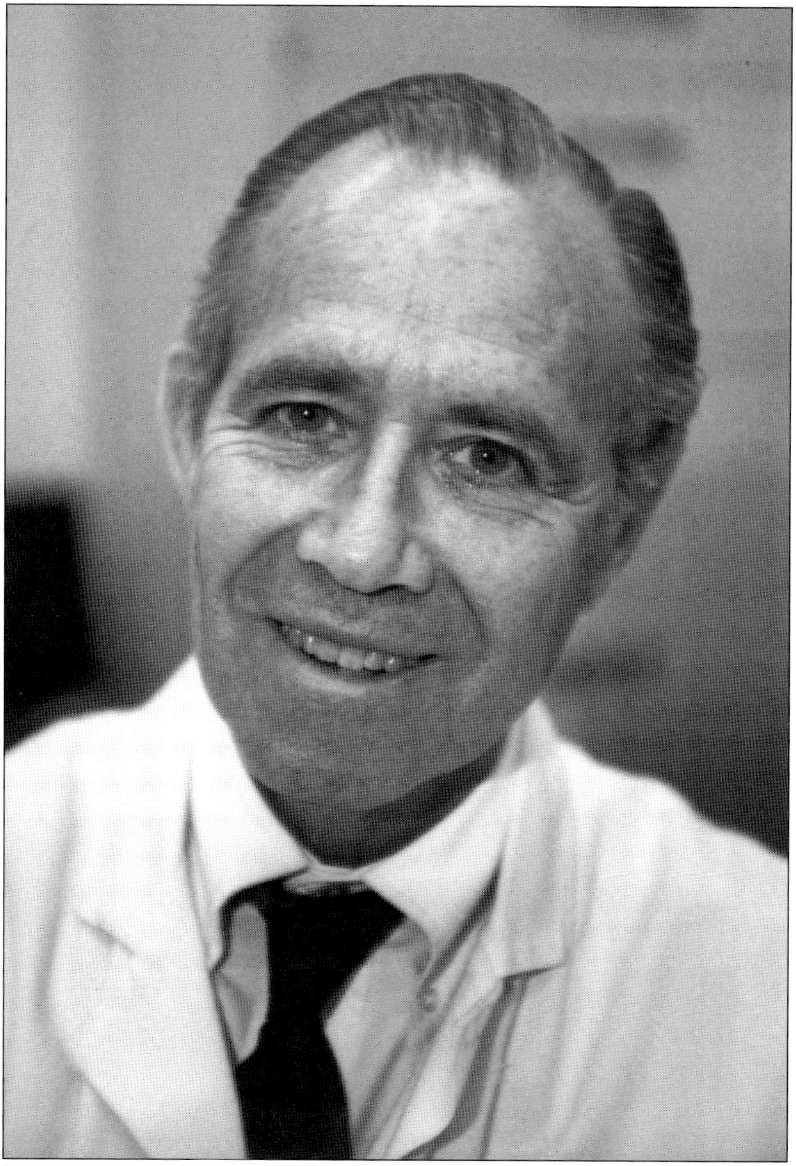

Robert Mellins was born in Brooklyn. He received a bachelor of arts degree from Columbia University and a medical degree from Johns Hopkins University. He completed residency training at the Babies Hospital and fellowship training in pediatrics, cardiology, and pulmonary medicine. Mellins joined the faculty at Columbia in 1957 and focused his research over the next five decades on the pathophysiology and clinical management of asthma. He became the first director of the Pediatric Pulmonary Division at Columbia's College of Physicians and Surgeons and is remembered as one of the founding fathers of the specialty of pediatric pulmonology. Mellins was a devoted physician, an inspiring mentor, and an international authority in the field of pediatric asthma. He received the Distinguished Service Award of the Columbia University Medical Center and the Distinguished Alumnus Award of the College of Physicians and Surgeons. Dr. Mellins served as president of the American Thoracic Society (ATS) in 1982–1983. As the first and only pediatrician to hold this position, he was honored with the Pediatric Assembly's Founders Award and later by the ATS Distinguished Achievement Award.

Five

The Modern Era

The modern era of the Babies Hospital is defined as the post-McIntosh period from 1960 through 2000. There were four Reuben S. Carpentier Professors and chairs of the department of pediatrics: Edward C. Curnen, Richard Behrman, Michael Katz, and John M. Driscoll Jr. The growth of pediatric subspecialties, many the first such newly created divisions in the United States, continued unabated. Leading them were James Wolff in pediatric hematology-oncology, Jerry Jacobs in rheumatology, Thomas Santulli in pediatric surgery, Sylvia Griffiths and Welton Gersony in pediatric cardiology, Robert Mellins in pulmonology, and Martin Nash in nephrology, to name but a few.

In 1968, the Babies Hospital doubled in size with the completion of the central building; the new addition added contemporary neonatal and critical care units, surgical operating rooms, and a radiology suite.

Babies Hospital clinicians and investigators continued their pursuit of discovery and innovation. New entities described include McCune-Albright syndrome, Kasbach-Merritt disease, shaken baby syndrome, and Riley-Day syndrome. In 1984, Dr. Eric Rose, a heart surgeon working with cardiologist Dr. Linda Addonizio, performed one of the earliest successful heart transplants in a child. In this period, the research of Dr. Anne Gershon was critical to the widespread adoption of the varicella vaccine, which prevents chickenpox.

In 2000, investment bank Morgan Stanley Dean Witter gifted NewYork-Presbyterian more than $55 million to build the Morgan Stanley Dean Witter Children's Hospital at 165th Street and Broadway to add to the Babies and Children's Hospital. In 2003, the name of the hospital was forever changed to the Morgan Stanley Children's Hospital of NewYork-Presbyterian.

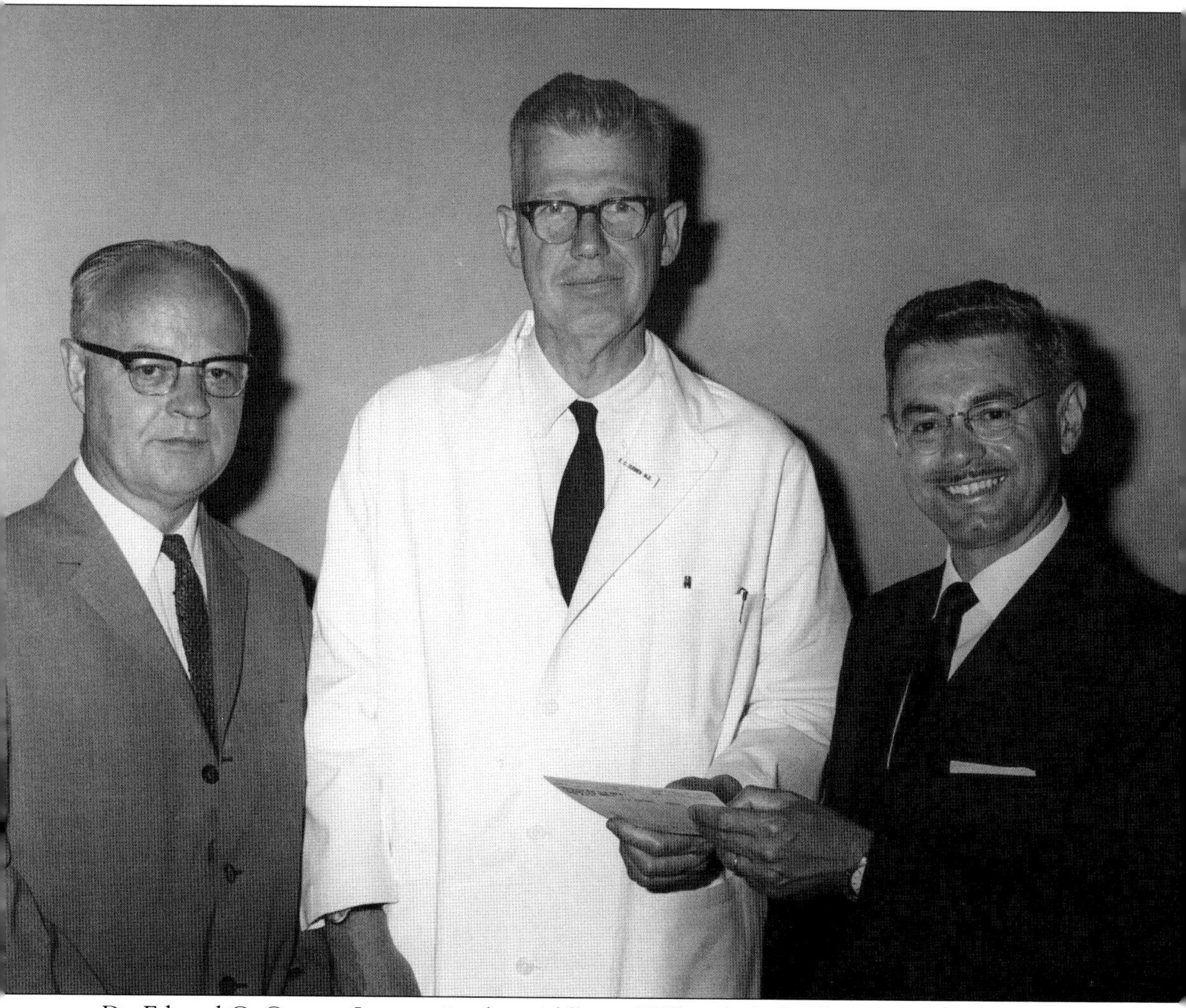

Dr. Edward C. Curnen Jr., seen in the middle in 1965 with Columbia medical school dean H. Houston Merritt (left) and a representative of Wyeth Laboratories, led Babies Hospital from 1960 to 1969 as director and chairman of pediatrics. Curnen was educated at Yale (AB, 1931) and Harvard (MD, 1935) and did a residency at Boston's Infants' and Children's Hospital. In 1939, he joined the Rockefeller Institute for Medical Research, where he did bacteriological studies with Oswald T. Avery and Colin M. McLeod. After wartime service, Curnen went to the Yale School of Medicine, where he researched polio, infectious mononucleosis, and dengue fever. In 1952, he became the first professor and chairman of the new department of pediatrics at the medical school of the University of North Carolina, Chapel Hill. Curnen's decade of service at Babies Hospital saw the construction of a major addition, Babies Hospital South, and the continued growth of pediatric subspecialties. In 1974, the hospital established the Edward C. Curnen Jr. Award to honor the pediatric resident who best exemplifies the humane and compassionate patient care characteristic of Dr. Curnen.

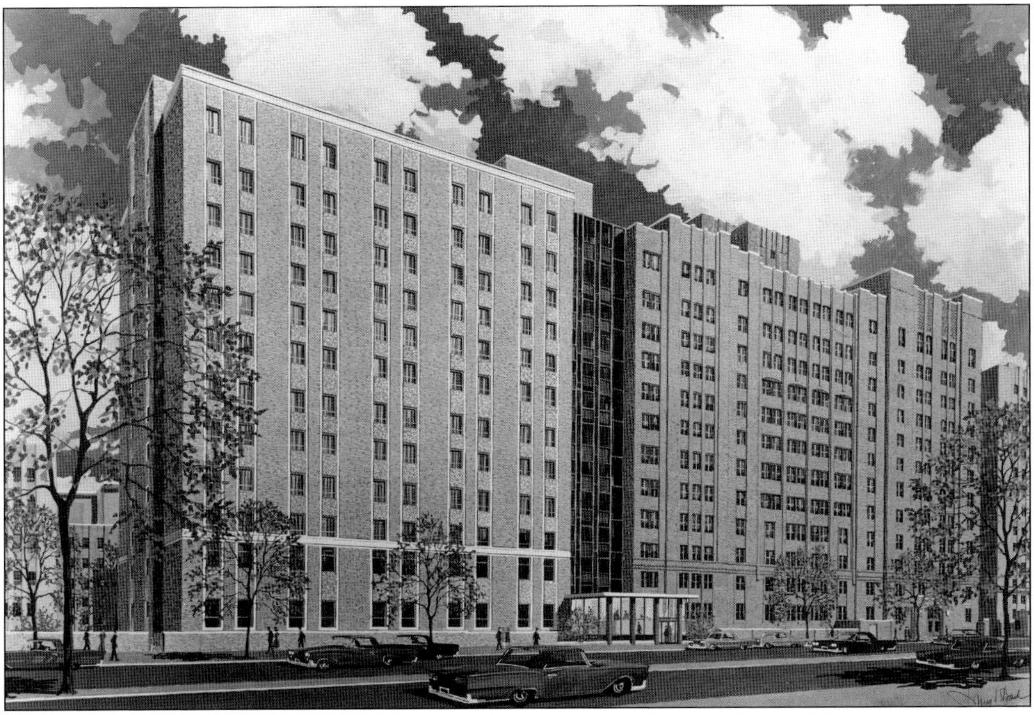

After more than 30 years in its 1929 home, Babies Hospital entered the 1960s with a structure that was overcrowded and out of date. A program of renovation and expansion began in 1966, when many laboratories moved to the recently completed William Black Research Building. At the same time, work began on what was then called Babies Hospital South (now known as Children's Hospital Central Building). The 12-story structure, seen above in an architectural rendering, was designed by Rogers, Butler & Burgun to harmonize with the original building. Funding was an issue, and at first, only four stories were completed—two basement levels and two above ground, as seen below in this December 1966 photograph. Work resumed in 1968 on the additional 10 stories, but even after completion in 1970, many floors remained unfinished. (Below, photograph by Elizabeth Wilcox.)

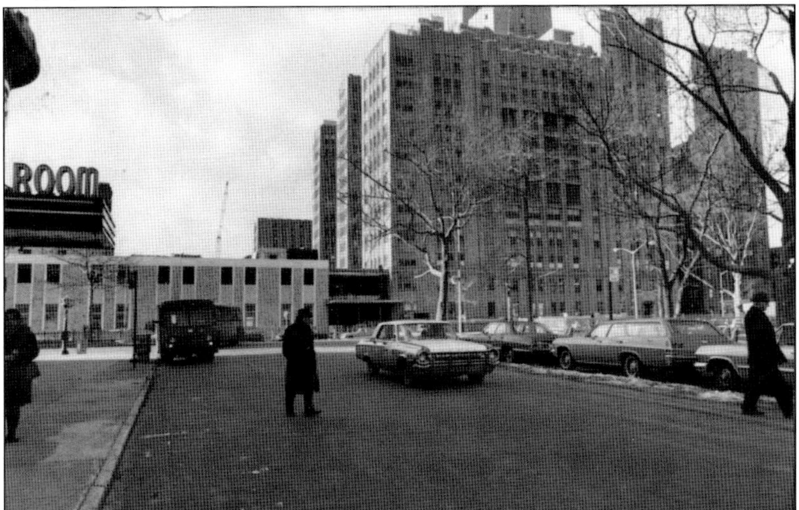

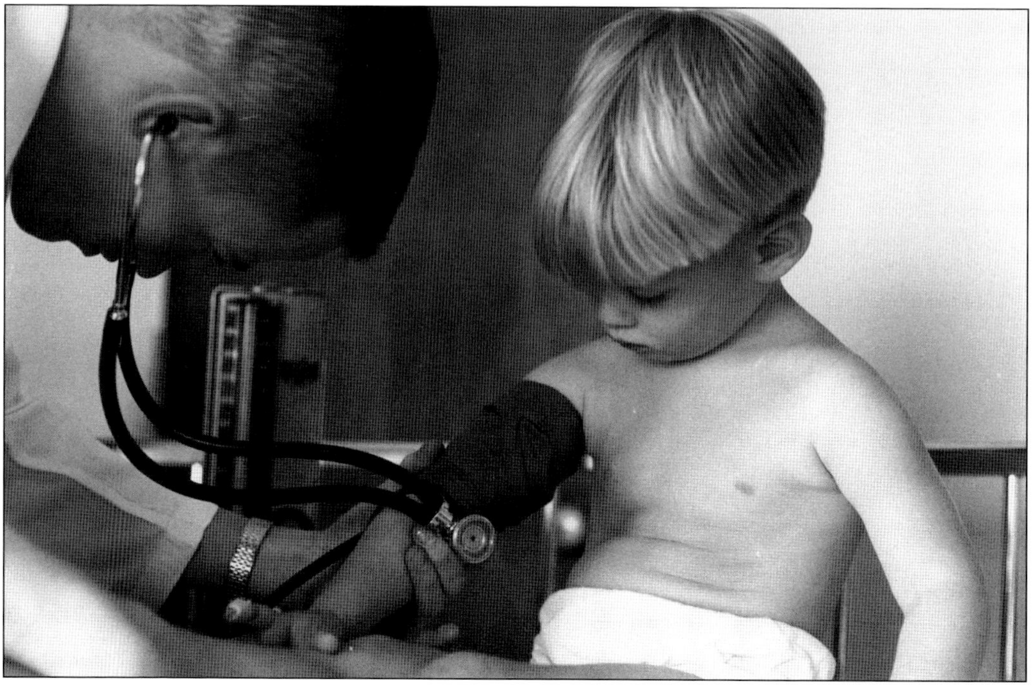

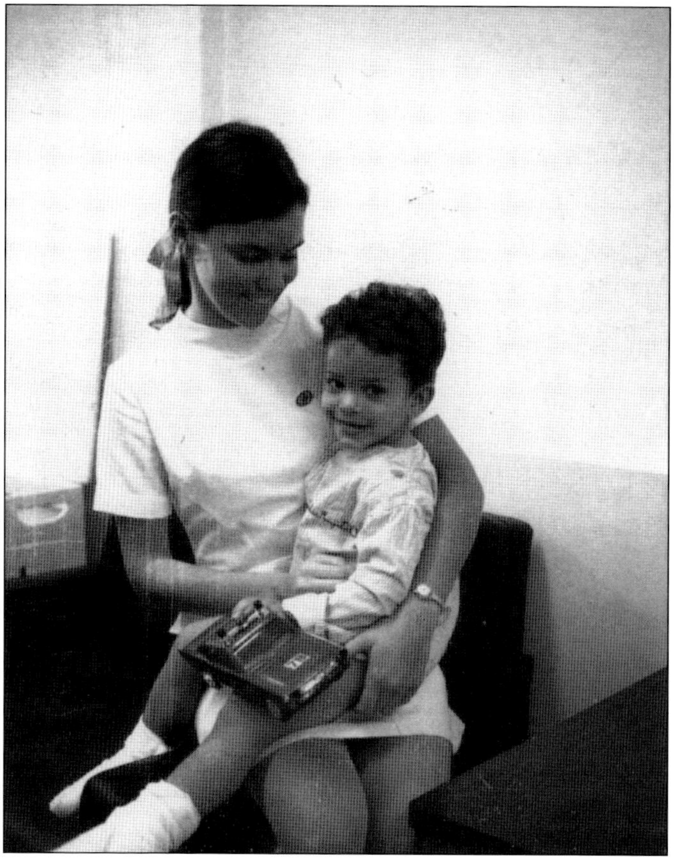

A resident takes Timmy's blood pressure at Babies Hospital in 1964. His story of having a tonsillectomy was the subject of a booklet covering everything a parent needed to know about their child's hospital stay from admission through discharge. Written in the form of a letter from one mother to another, it was illustrated with images taken by the medical center's talented photographer, Elizabeth Wilcox. (Photograph by Elizabeth Wilcox.)

It was "Christmas in July" when the Children's Christmas Fund of New York City radio station WOR made a generous donation of gifts for Babies Hospital patients in July 1972. Seen here is nurse Mary Giovanelli holding a little patient happily grasping his new present: a toy car. (Photograph by Lucy Lazzopina.)

The first Children's Heart Day was held at the hospital in May 1973 to highlight the success of its pediatric open-heart surgery program. The reunion was attended by about 250 of the more than 1,000 children who in the past decade had the operation at Babies Hospital. They were hailed as "medical pioneers" who had helped make open-heart surgery a safer, more common procedure. To the right, Dr. James Malm, director of pediatric open-heart surgery, welcomed the guests and announced the formation of the Children's Heart Club, a volunteer organization to support the hospital's heart center. Among the guests were baseball legends Tom Seaver and Willie Mays (below) of the New York Mets, who chatted with the children and signed autographs. Children and parents then left for Shea Stadium to see the Mets play the Pittsburgh Pirates.

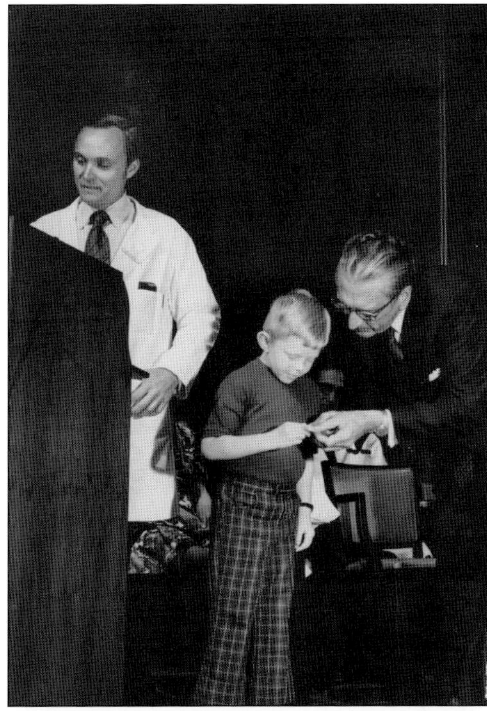

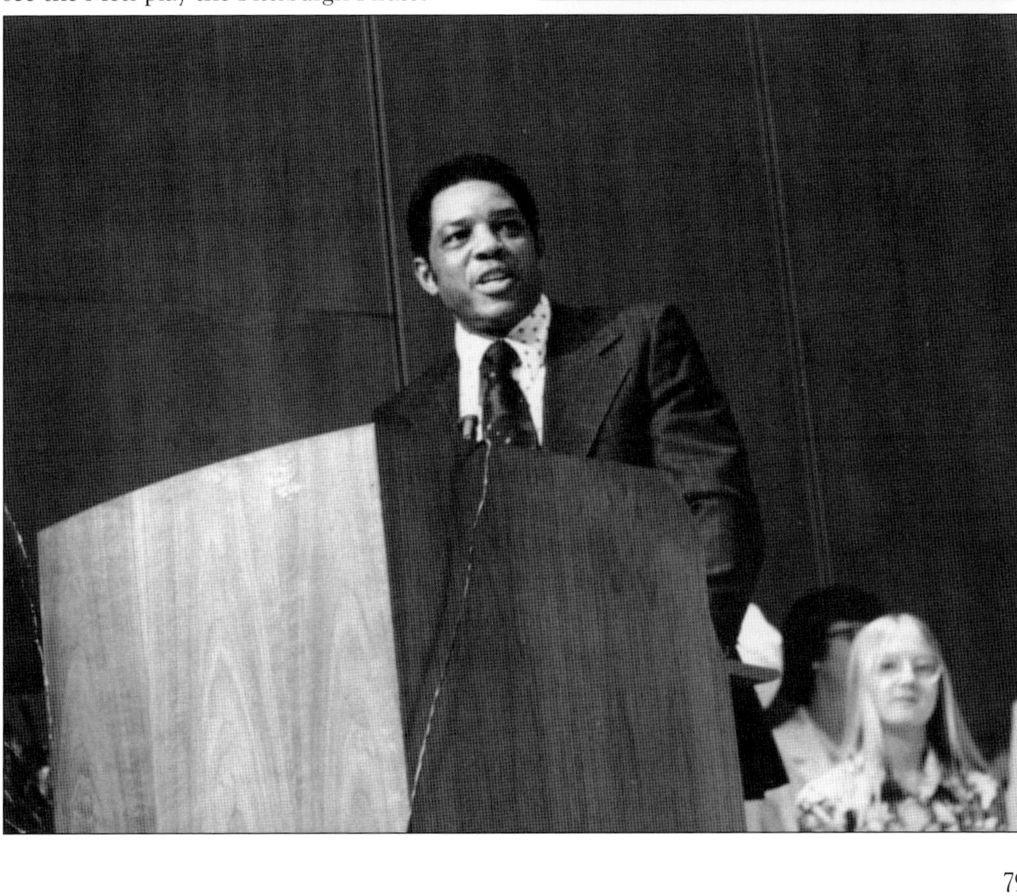

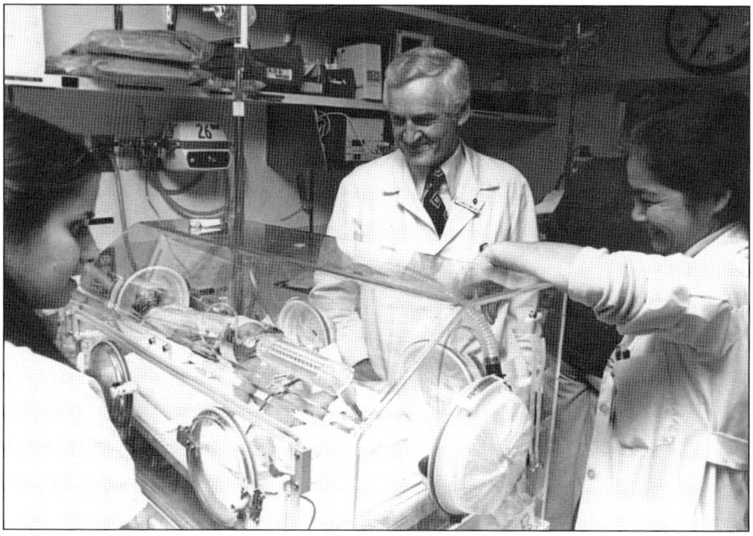

L. Stanley James is seen here in the neonatal intensive care unit at Babies Hospital with a premature infant, probably sometime in the 1980s. The New Zealand–born James is considered one of the founders of perinatology and spent much of his 40 years at the hospital heading its division of perinatal medicine. (Photograph by Arthur Pease.)

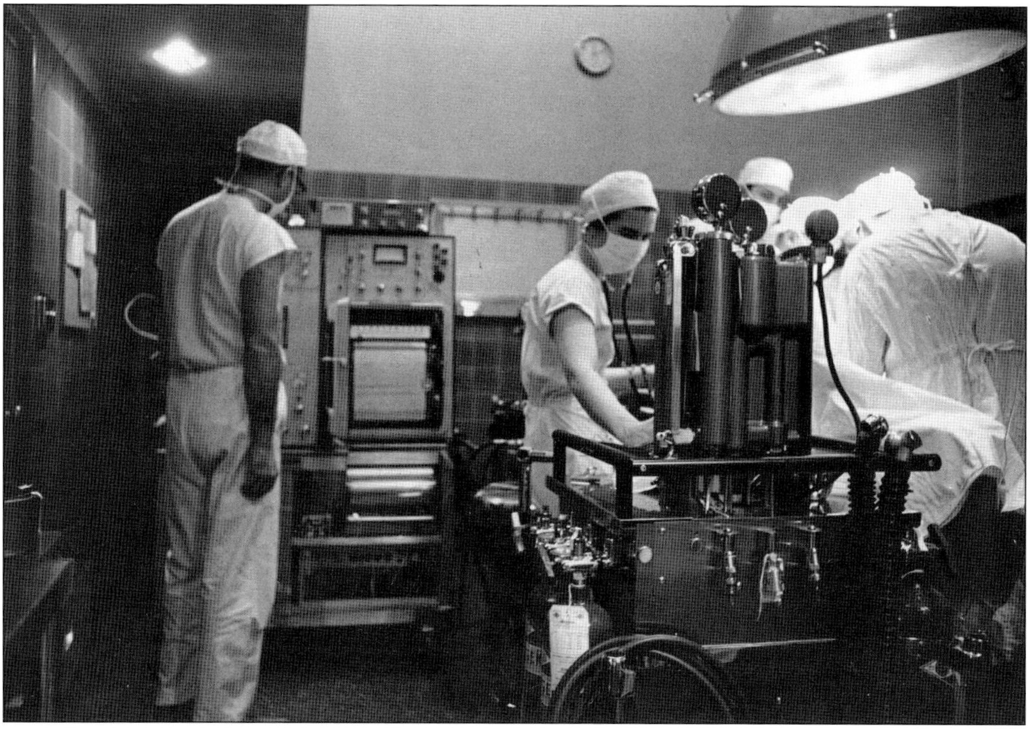

Anesthesiologist Herbert Rackow, seen at left, monitors readings during surgery in a Babies Hospital operating room in 1964. Rackow and his hospital colleague, Ernest Salanitre, were among the founders of pediatric anesthesiology in the 1950s–1960s. Their 1969 article "Modern Concepts in Pediatric Anesthesiology" is considered a landmark in the field, and they were among the founders of the Section on Anesthesiology of the American Academy of Pediatrics. (Photograph by Elizabeth Wilcox.)

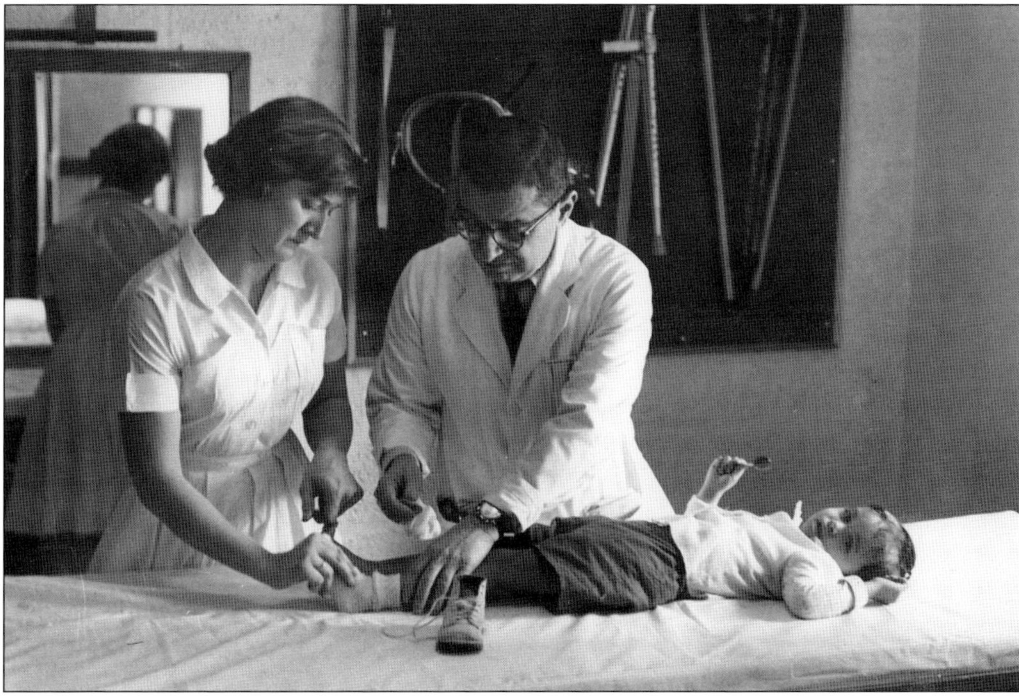

Dr. Milton Singer examines a patient with the assistance of a physical therapist at the Babies Hospital Cerebral Palsy Clinic in 1963. The patient, pacified with a lollipop, seems more interested in the photographer. Singer was then engaged in a collaborative research effort with the medical center's department of orthopedic surgery to determine how effective surgical intervention might be in alleviating the symptoms of the disease. (Photograph by Elizabeth Wilcox.)

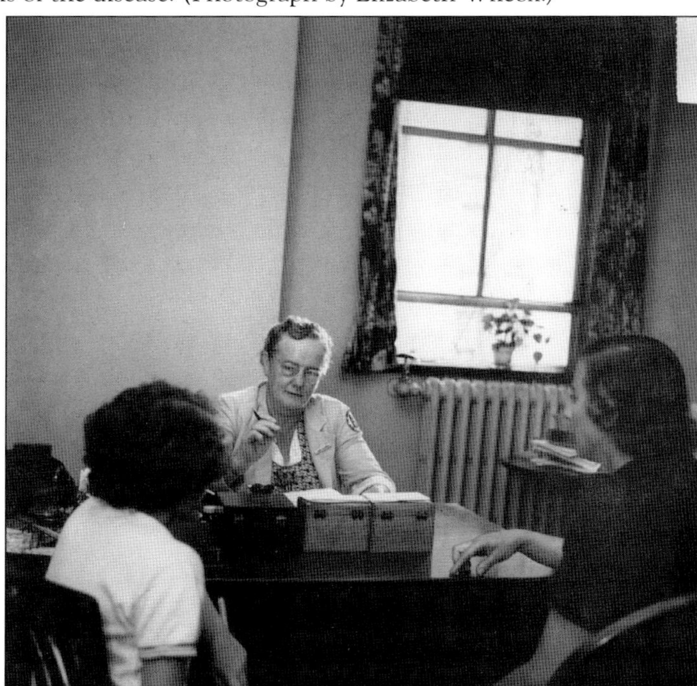

Pediatric social worker Adelaide Vrooman interviews a patient and mother in 1965. Social work at Babies Hospital dates to the early 1900s, when it first employed a visiting nurse. By the 1920s, it had a full social work department offering many services to families. Babies Hospital's social work retained its separate identity until 1955, when all social work at the medical center was consolidated into one department. (Photograph by Elizabeth Wilcox.)

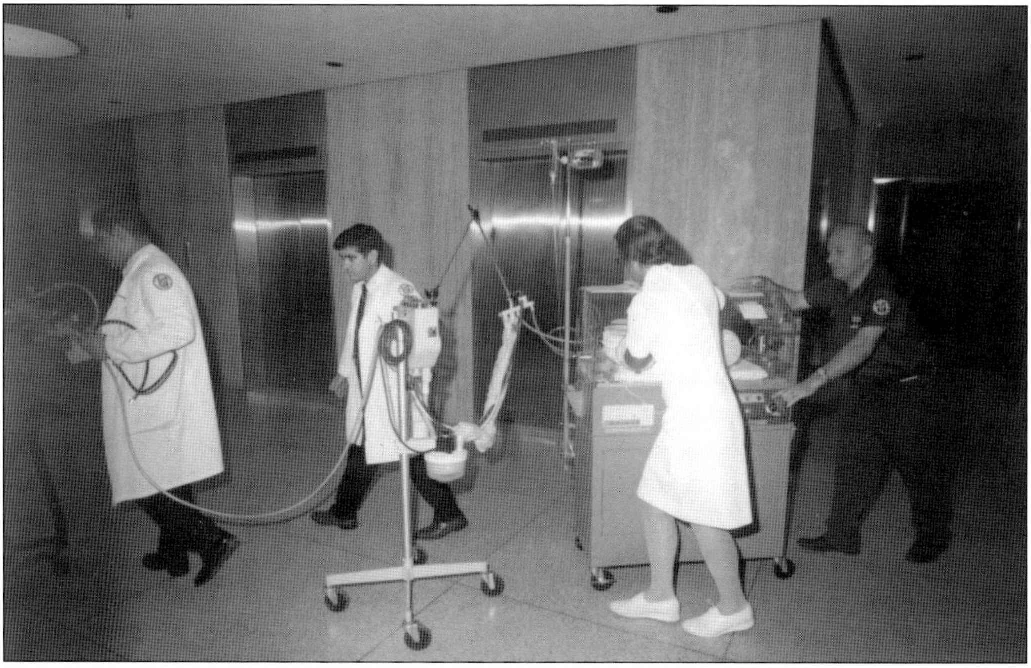

Shortly before 4:00 a.m. on August 5, 1969, a fire broke out in a nurses' classroom on the second floor of Babies Hospital. Located just about 30 yards down the corridor from the fire was the Neonatal Intensive Care Unit (NICU), whose 22 infants would have been severely affected by even a trace of smoke. While the New York City Fire Department was called immediately, it was the quick action of hospital personnel including security officers, residents, and maintenance workers that prevented a tragedy by quickly evacuating the infants' isolettes to a safe location. Subsequent examination determined that none had suffered from smoke inhalation. The fire was confined to the classroom, and two days later, the isolettes with their precious occupants were able to be returned to the NICU by hospital staff, as seen in these photographs.

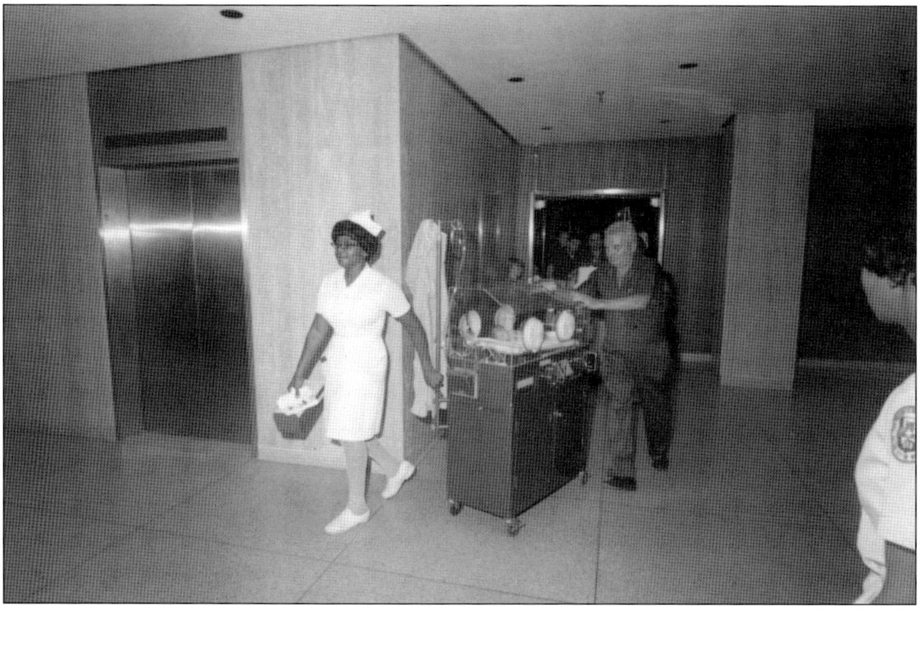

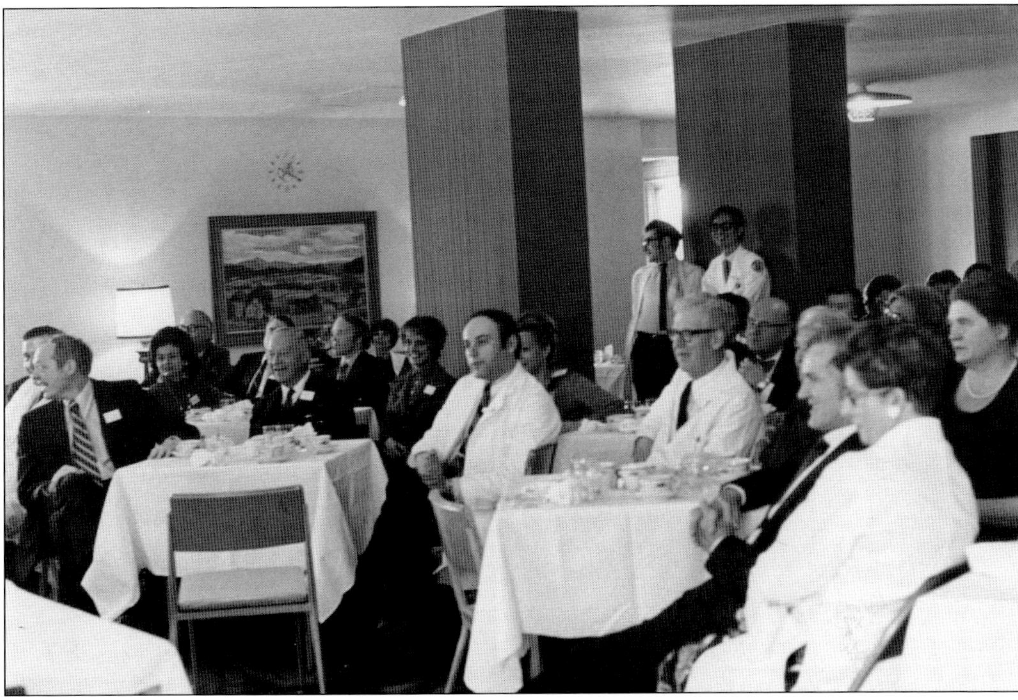

Members of the Babies Hospital Alumni Association listen to a presentation at the annual reunion in April 1972 (above). Forming an alumni association was first discussed in 1927, but the organization was not formally founded until 1937. Its mission, as stated by Babies Hospital director Herbert B. Wilcox in the hospital's 1927 annual report, was to "keep alive the interest of our graduates and attract new men [*sic*] to us." The alumni association supports that mission by sponsoring yearly meetings featuring scholarly lectures on a variety of medical and scientific topics. Perhaps its most important role is to renew the bonds forged among the interns and residents while they were serving in the hospital. At right, from left to right, Drs. L. Stanley James, Katherine Merritt, and Richard E. Behrman catch up during the reunion's luncheon in April 1972.

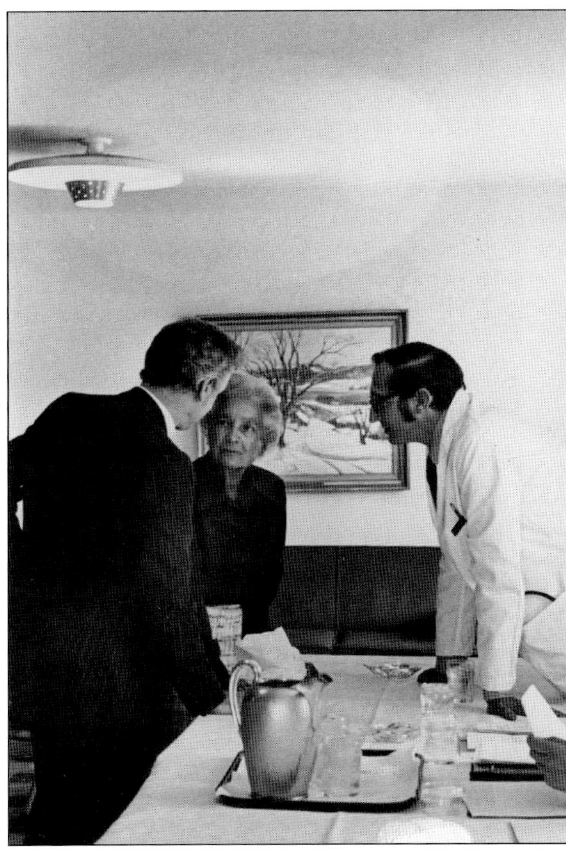

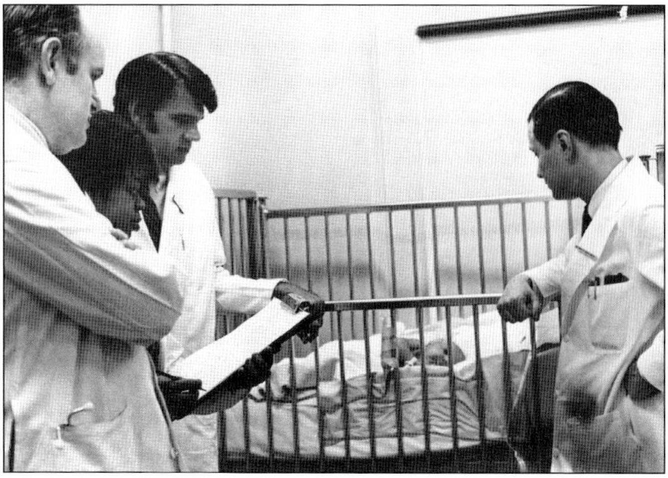

This concerned group is gathered around a patient who is being fed intravenously. In 1972, a team of physicians at Babies Hospital, headed by Thomas Santulli and Robert Winters, led a major National Institutes of Health–funded research effort to study ways of improving intravenous feeding of infants. Seen here, from left to right, are John M. Driscoll, Constance Rochester, RN, William C. Heird, and John N. Schullinger. (Photograph by Lucy Lazzopina.)

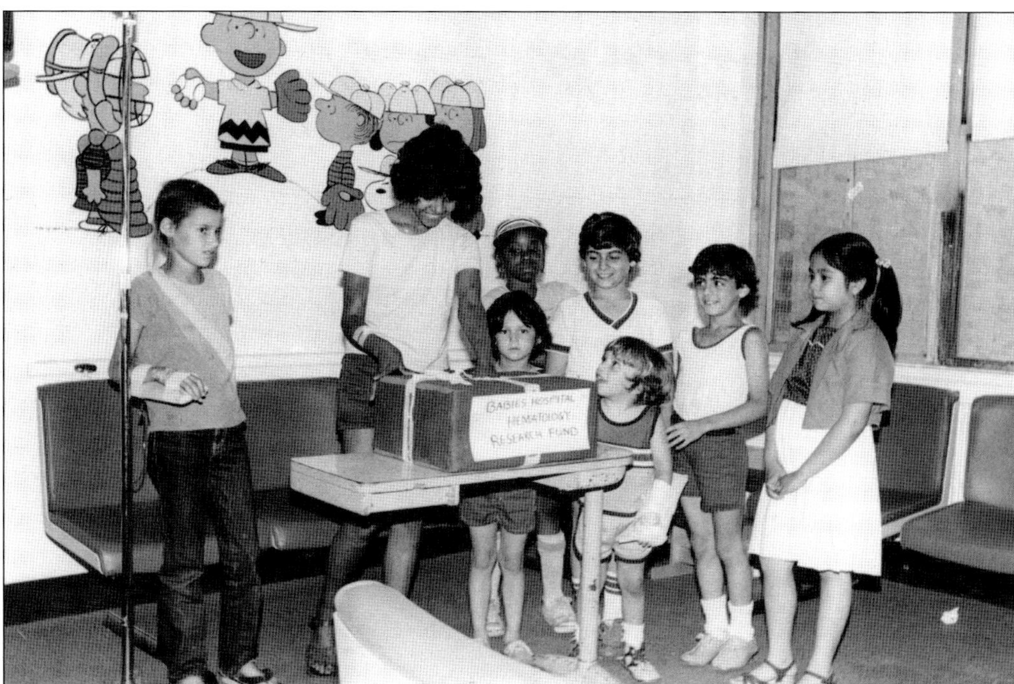

A patient prepares to pick the winners in the raffle organized on behalf of the children aided by the Babies Hospital Hematology Research Fund while other patients and their family members look on in 1980. Medical center publications at the time noted that the raffle had been a huge success with several thousand tickets sold and thanked the parents of the pediatric hematology patients for organizing it.

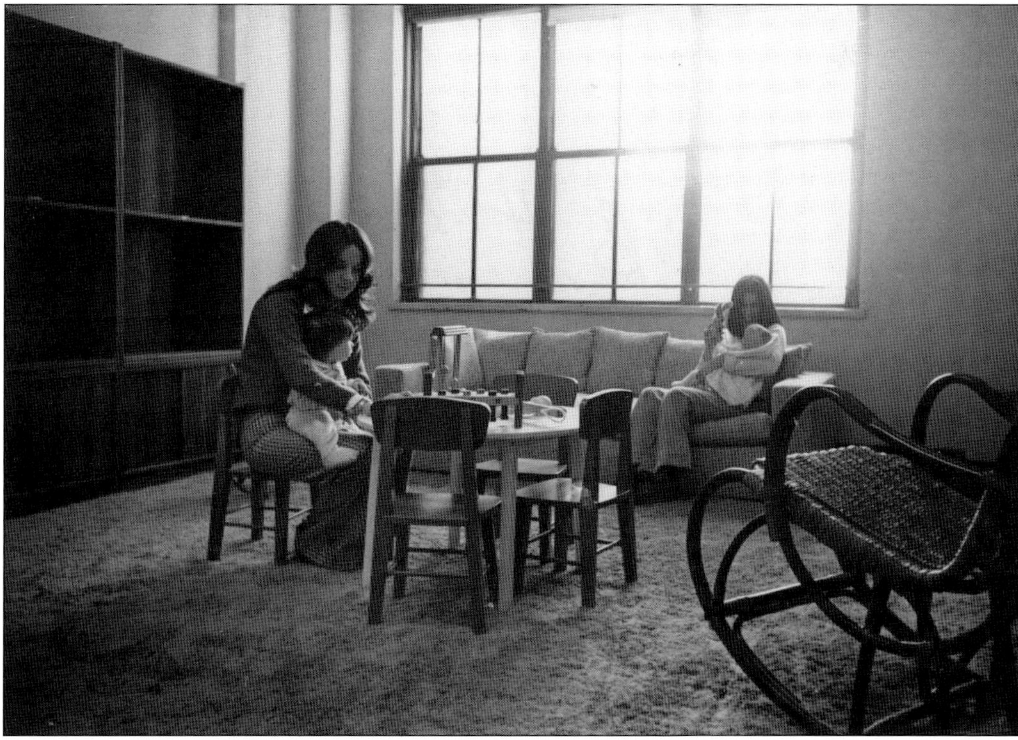

Many children's hospitals have parenting rooms, but few if any have been furnished by New York's famed Bloomingdale's department store. Seen here are two mothers visiting their recently hospitalized children in a newly created visiting room for parents in 1976. Located on Babies Hospital's eighth floor, the space had originally been a storage room. Bloomingdale's helped with the design and then generously donated the furnishings as well.

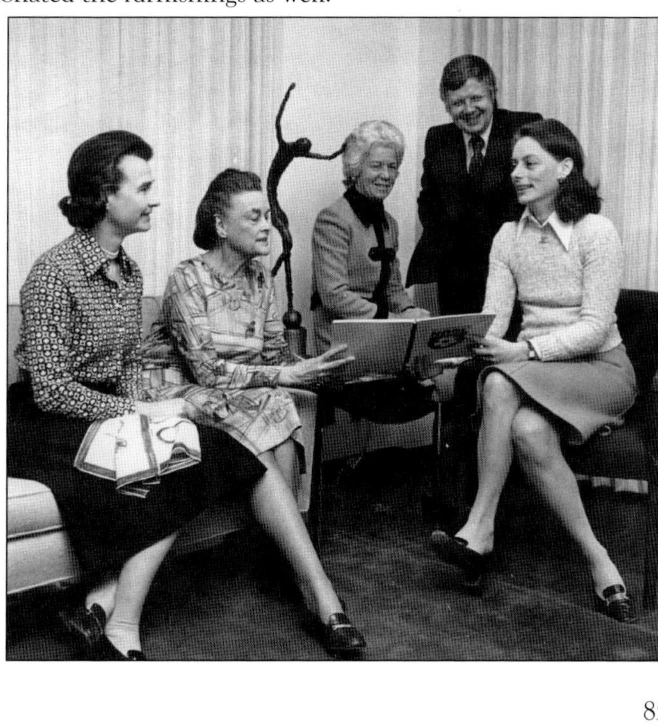

Members of the Babies Hospital Board of Women Managers gather to plan "A Celebrity Soccer Night" benefit to see the renowned superstar Pelé play with the New York Cosmos in 1976. Seated from left to right are Mary Braga, Jane E. Hill, Emily Tucker, and Marion H.C. Bedrick; behind them is Clive Toye, general manager of the Cosmos. The board was Babies Hospital's long-standing fund-raising arm.

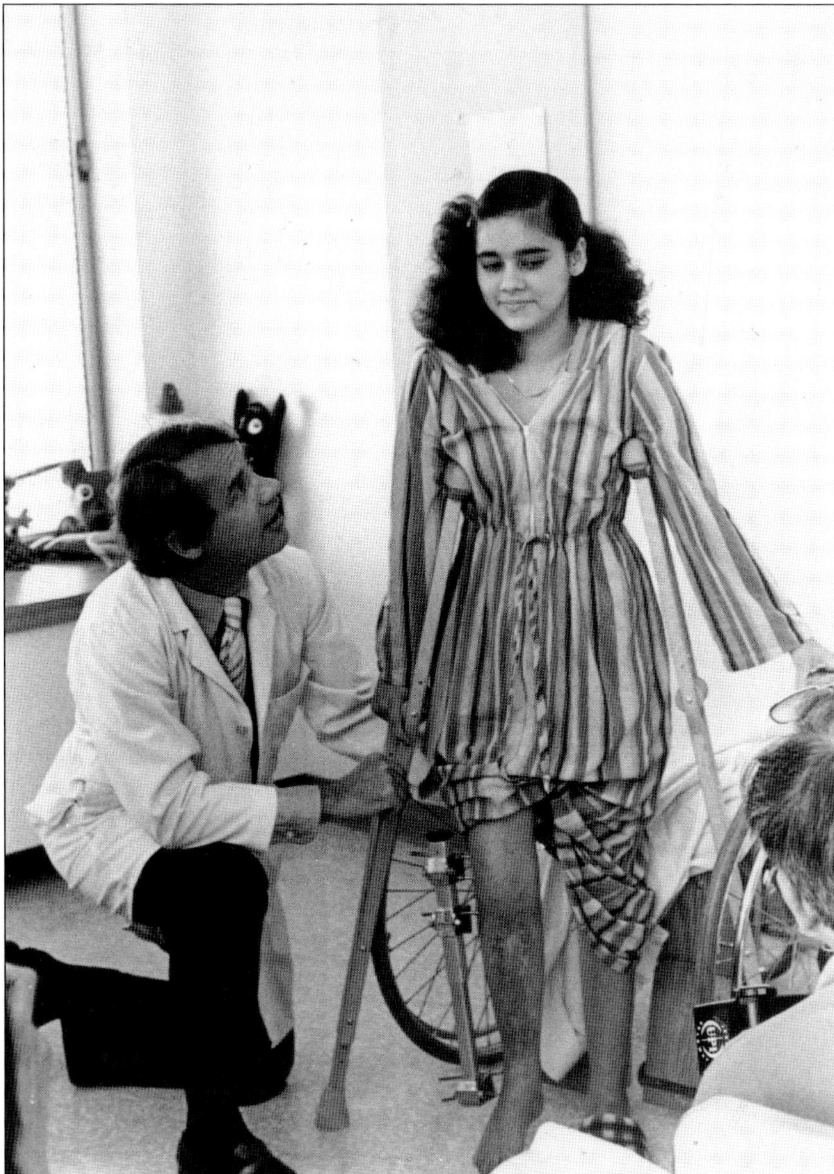

Dr. Harold Dick, chief of the Columbia-Presbyterian Medical Center's Orthopedic Pediatric Service, examines the leg of a young patient in 1979. Harold Dick, a native New Yorker, graduated from Princeton University and New York University School of Medicine. He completed his orthopedic residency at the Columbia-Presbyterian Medical Center. Dr. Dick completed two fellowships, with one in hand surgery at Columbia and the second in orthopedic oncology at the Memorial Sloan Kettering Cancer Center. He joined the Columbia faculty in 1969 and served as chair of the department of orthopedics from 1984 to 1998. During his tenure, he developed the center for orthopedic research, as well as centers of excellence in microsurgery, trauma, and sports medicine. He helped pioneer limb-sparing techniques, including allograft, autograft, and fibular transplants and limb-lengthening procedures for the surgical management of patients with cancer of the upper and lower extremities. Dr. Dick had a special rapport with pediatric patients that provided compassion and comfort under difficult circumstances.

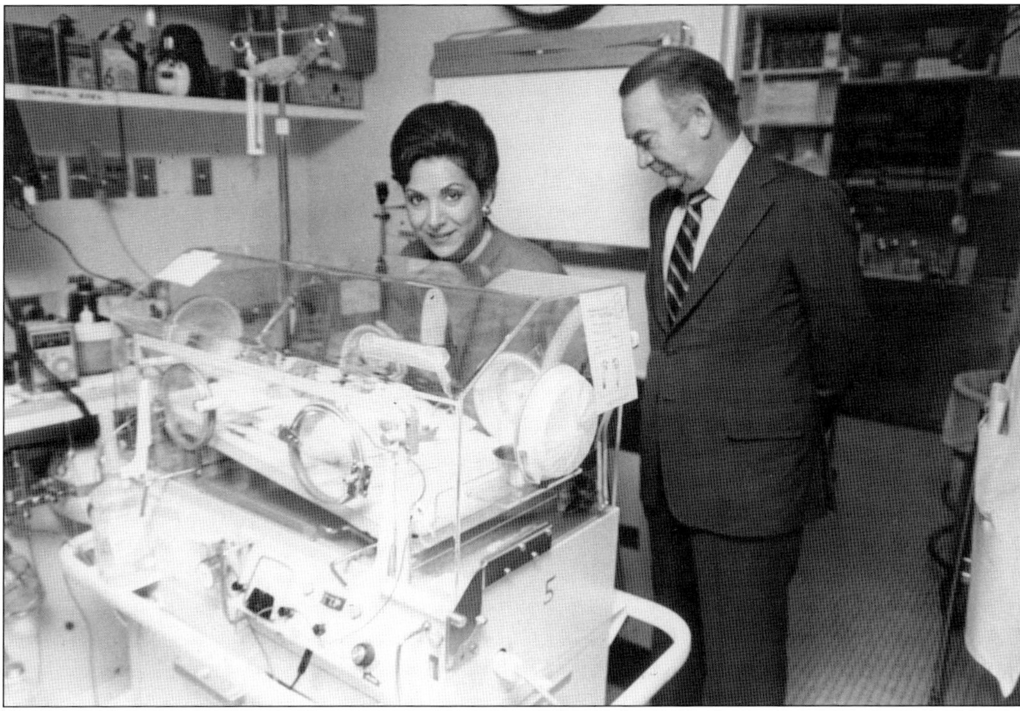

Besides entertainers, many political figures have trekked to Babies Hospital over the years. Above, New York governor Hugh Carey and his wife, Evangeline Gouletas Carey, are seen in the Neonatal Intensive Care Unit in June 1982. They were there to draw attention to a task force headed by Evangeline on the role of nutrition in New York State. Below, Madeleine Albright, then US ambassador to the United Nations and later the first female US secretary of state, visits the hospital in 1993 as part of President Clinton's health reform efforts. She is seen with Babies Hospital director and chairman of pediatrics John Driscoll (second from left) and Allen Hyman, Presbyterian Hospital chief of staff and professor of anesthesiology (second from right). (Below, photograph by Leslie Bernstein.)

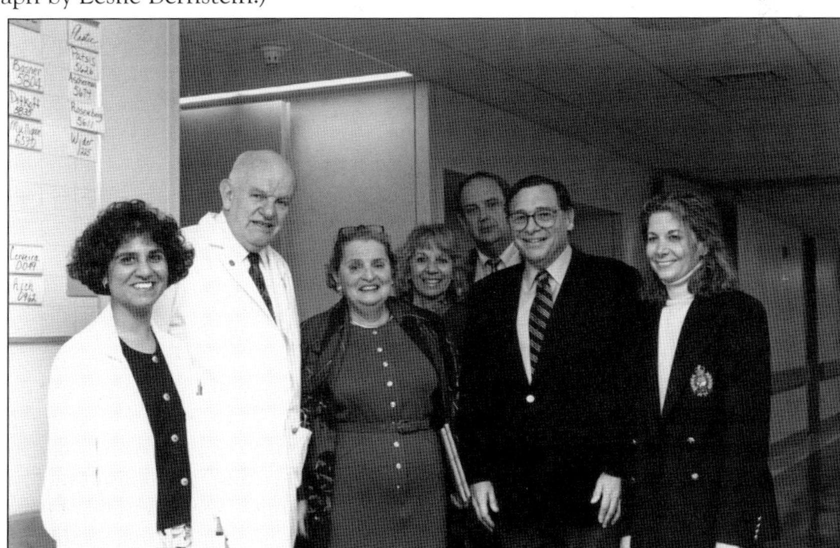

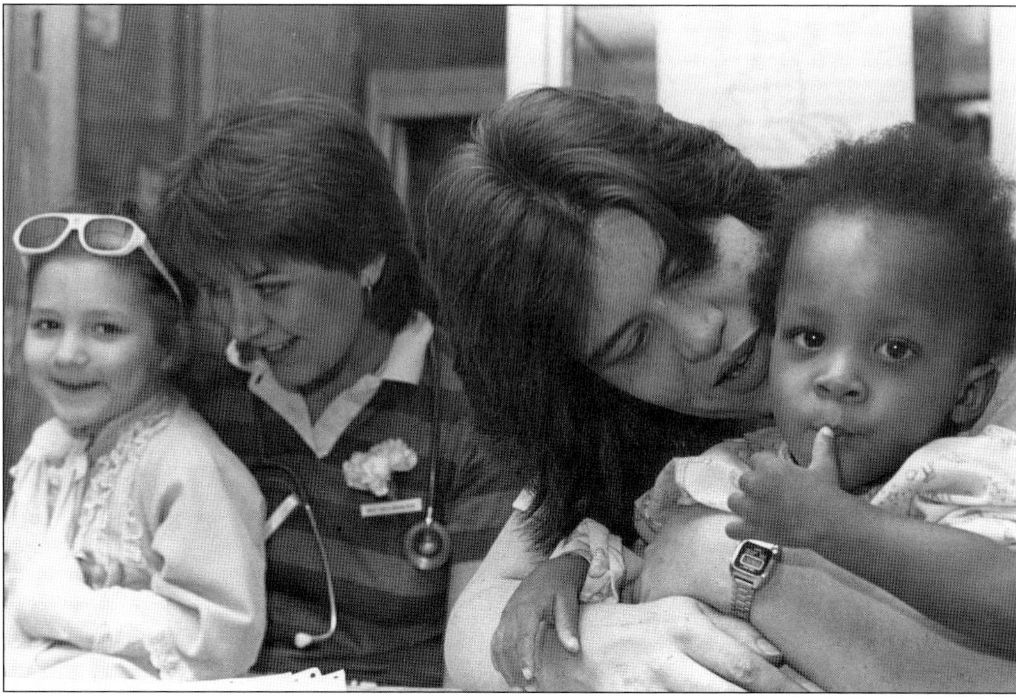

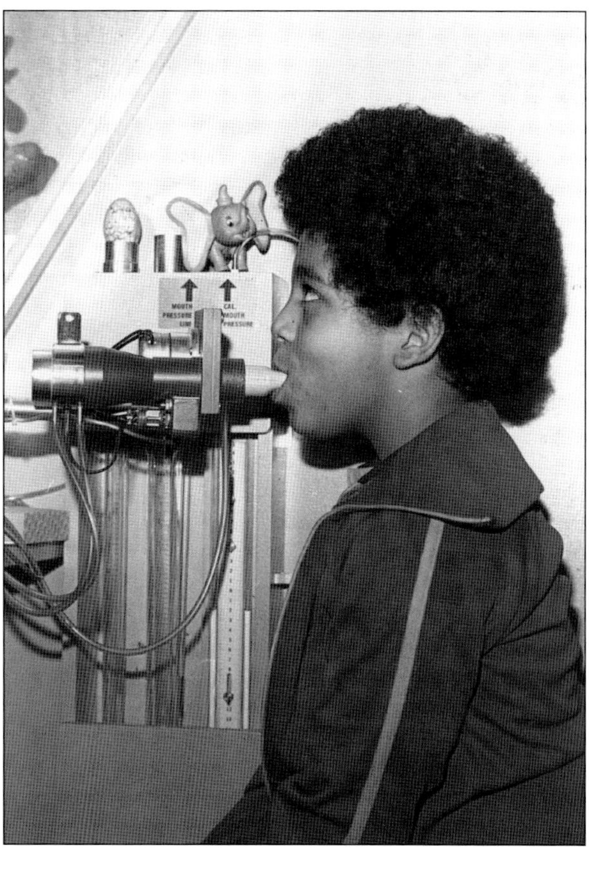

Nurses Meg Halloran (left) and Jeanne Figueira (right) attend to their patients at Babies Hospital in 1983. They were part of the new Center for Women and Children, which brought together pediatricians and obstetricians to provide seamless care for mother and child at the time of delivery. Newborns needing immediate medical care could be quickly transferred to the intensive care unit, located on the same floor as the delivery rooms.

A young patient takes a pulmonary function test in 1983. Under Dr. Robert Mellins, director of the pediatric pulmonary division, Babies Hospital became a center of excellence for the treatment of children's lung diseases. The division saw children with asthma and cystic fibrosis, as well as those with pulmonary complications due to orthopedic conditions such as curvature of the spine.

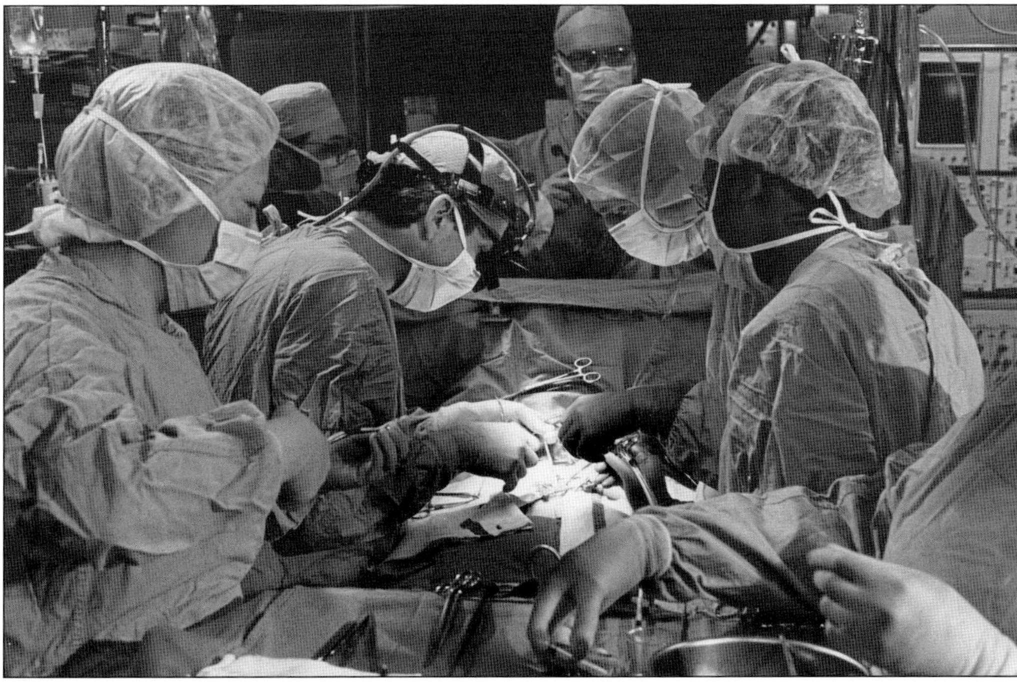

While Babies Hospital did not perform the first pediatric heart transplant, it was a pioneer in the field. Early attempts at heart transplants in children were not encouraging, with most recipients dying within a few hours. So when four-year-old J.P. Lovette entered Babies Hospital in 1984 for a transplant to cure a serious heart malformation, the odds for success were not good. On June 9 of that year, a surgical team led by Eric Rose performed Babies Hospital's first pediatric heart transplant. Seen in the photograph above is Rose on the left, wearing magnifying glasses to better see the tiny heart. The operation was a success, and Lovette, seen below with his parents after the operation, lived to be 25, dying in his sleep during his first week in medical school. (Above, photograph by Jeff Szmulewicz.)

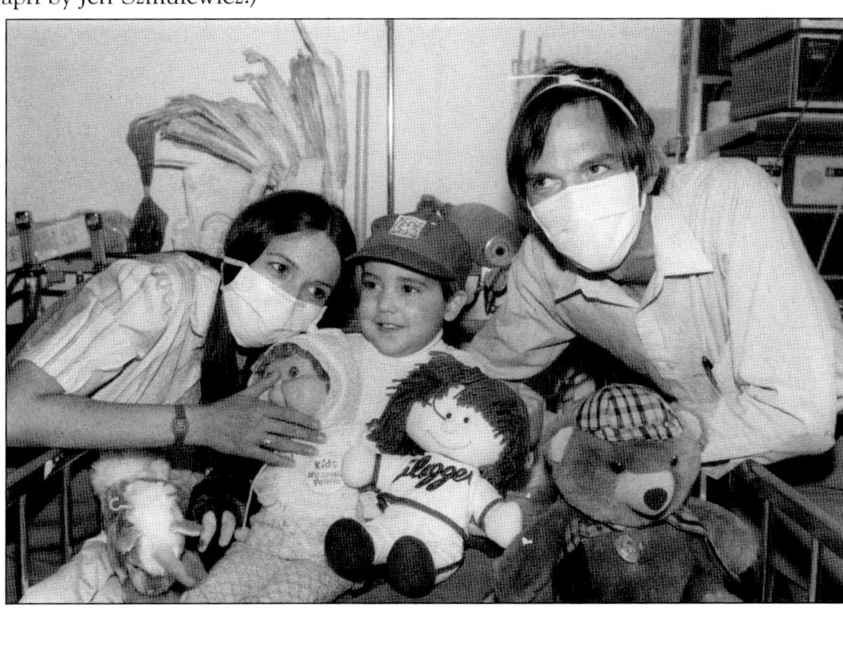

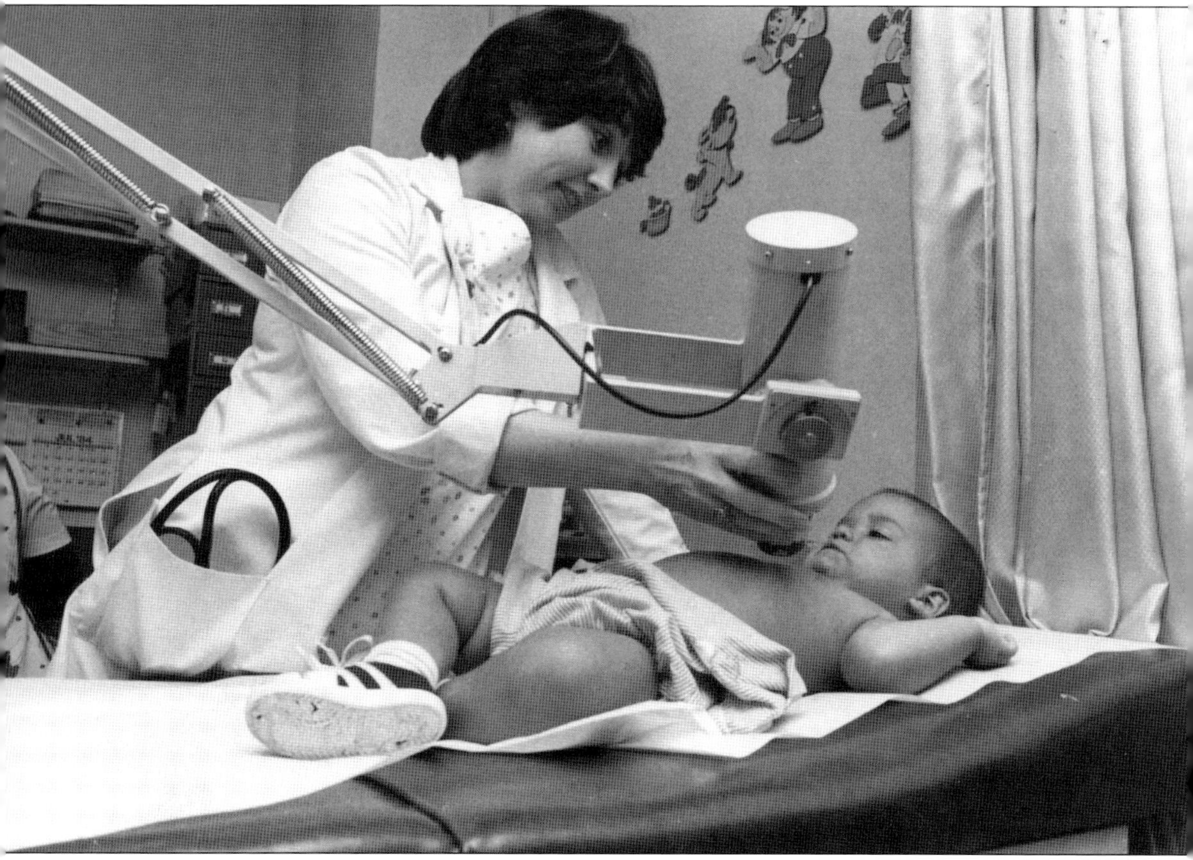

Linda Addonizio examines a young patient using a nuclear stethoscope in 1984. At the time the latest in medical technology, the nuclear stethoscope came equipped with its own computer, allowing physicians to measure heart function without having to do a lengthy and invasive cardiac catheterization. Addonizio, the James R. Malm, MD, Professor of Pediatric Cardiovascular Medicine, completed her undergraduate degree at Stanford University and graduated from the College of Physicians and Surgeons at Columbia University. She completed her residency and fellowship at the Babies Hospital and joined the faculty in the division of pediatric cardiology, where she remained her entire career. Dr. Addonizio established the cardiomyopathy and heart failure program and was instrumental in advancing child and adolescent heart transplantation, a program she founded and led for more than 35 years. The many honors and accolades accorded Dr. Addonizio include the Rustin McIntosh Award, the Governor's Award for Excellence as a Woman in History, and election to the Board of Directors of the International Society of Heart and Lung Transplantation.

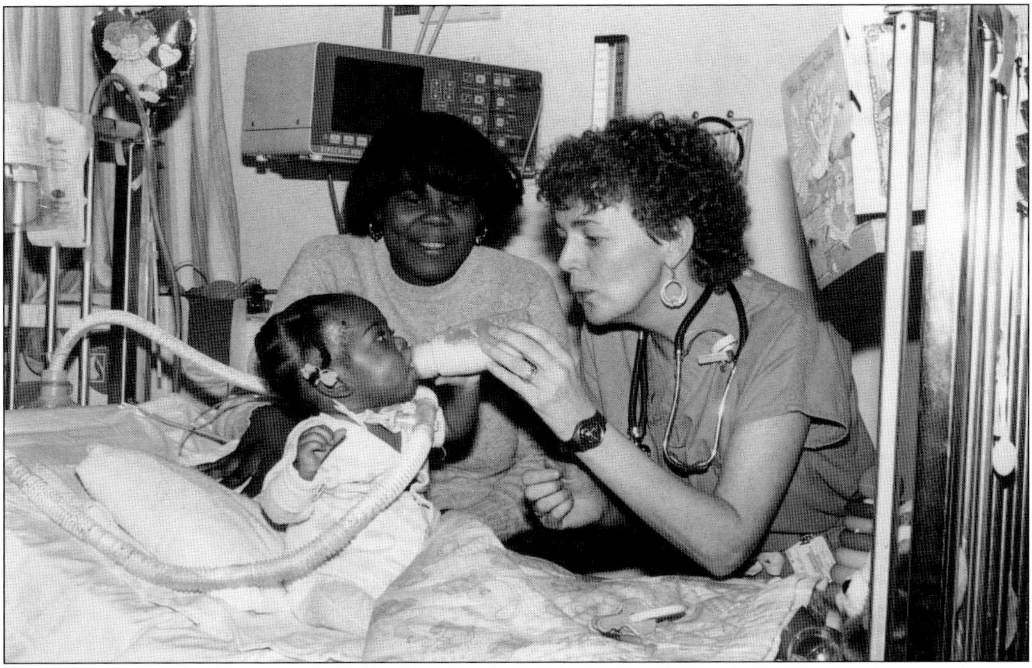

Judy Douglas, RN, feeds a one-year-old patient in the Babies Hospital Pediatric Intensive Care Unit (PICU) while the child's mother looks on in 1985. The PICU is where older children recover from surgery, and nursing care is crucial for the patients' return to health. As Douglas noted in the medical center's publication, the *Stethoscope*, at the time, "Minute-by-minute nursing observation is paramount to each child's care." (Photograph by Constance Grzelka.)

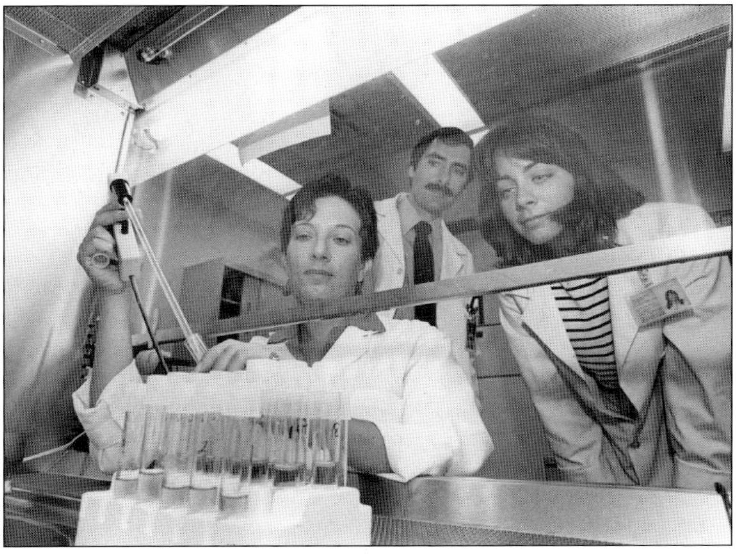

Research has a long history at Babies Hospital dating back to L. Emmett Holt's studies on infant feeding. Here, William Maltese, a cell biologist at the hospital's pediatric neurology divisional laboratory, oversees an experiment on cholesterol synthesis in 1985. Laboratory technician Ellen Tress is at left, while colleague Kathy Sheridan looks on. (Photograph by Joel Landau)

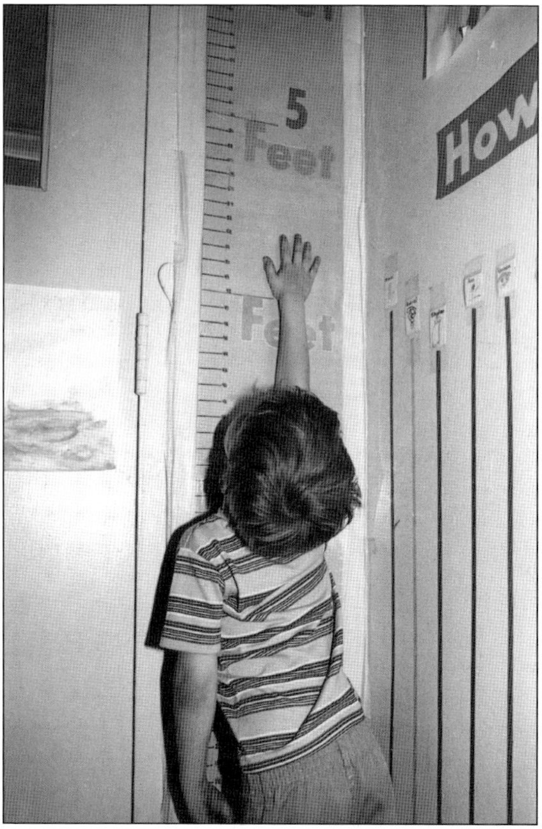

A child reaches for, if not the stars, at least a normal height in 1986. That year, Babies Hospital was given permission to begin using synthetic growth hormone on children whose physical growth would have been severely retarded otherwise. Previously, such children were treated with natural growth hormone, but possible side effects led the National Institutes of Health to prohibit its use in 1985. (Photograph by Gary Goldenberg.)

Thomas Q. Morris, president of Presbyterian Hospital, cuts the ribbon celebrating the opening of the fourth-floor addition to Babies Hospital in July 1987. The new space included state-of-the-art operating and recovery rooms, a therapeutic play space, and waiting rooms. Flanking Morris are, from left to right, R. Peter Altman, director of pediatric surgery; Carmela Grande, chief operating room nurse; Laura Flanagan, nurse; and Peter Rothstein, director of pediatric anesthesiology.

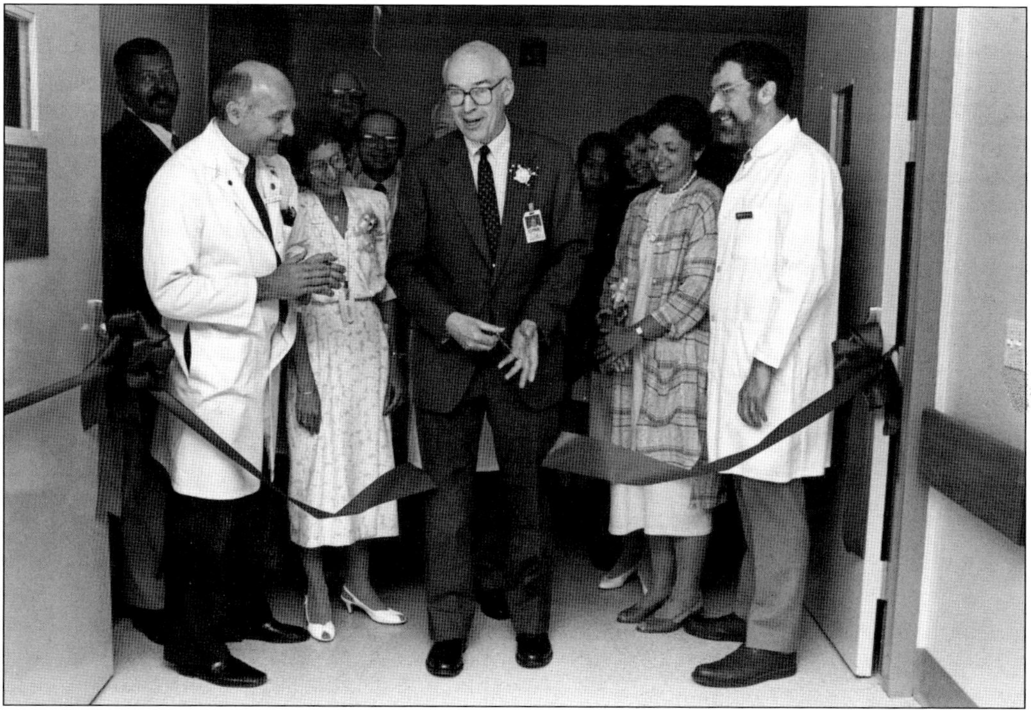

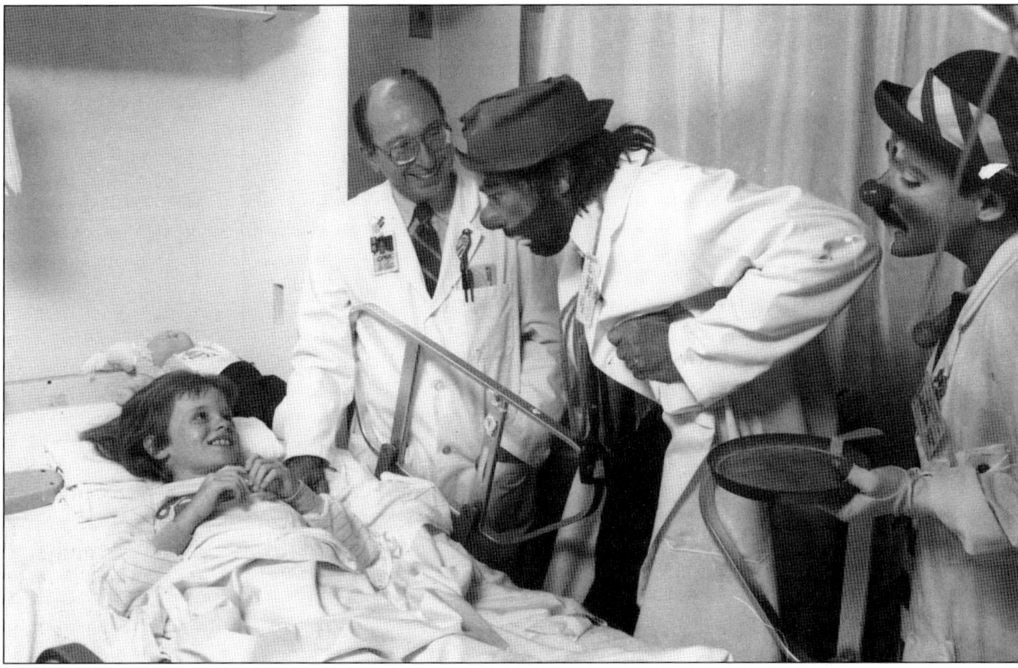

Clowns and children's hospitals are a perfect match, and over the years, Babies Hospital has had visits from many. Here, clowns from the Big Apple Circus interact with a young patient as part of a program called Clowns on Call in 1987. The initiative was launched to help children develop a positive attitude toward their illness.

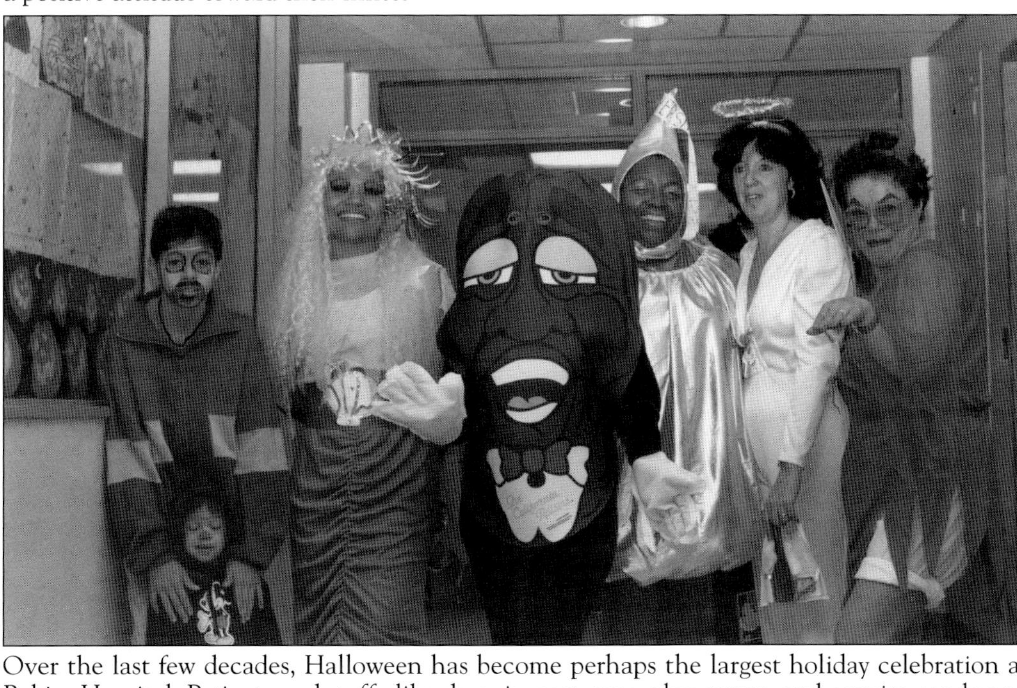

Over the last few decades, Halloween has become perhaps the largest holiday celebration at Babies Hospital. Patients and staff alike dress in costumes, play games, and acquire candy and toys. Here, staff members and what looks like at least one patient roam a hallway dressed in scary and not-so-scary costumes in 1991.

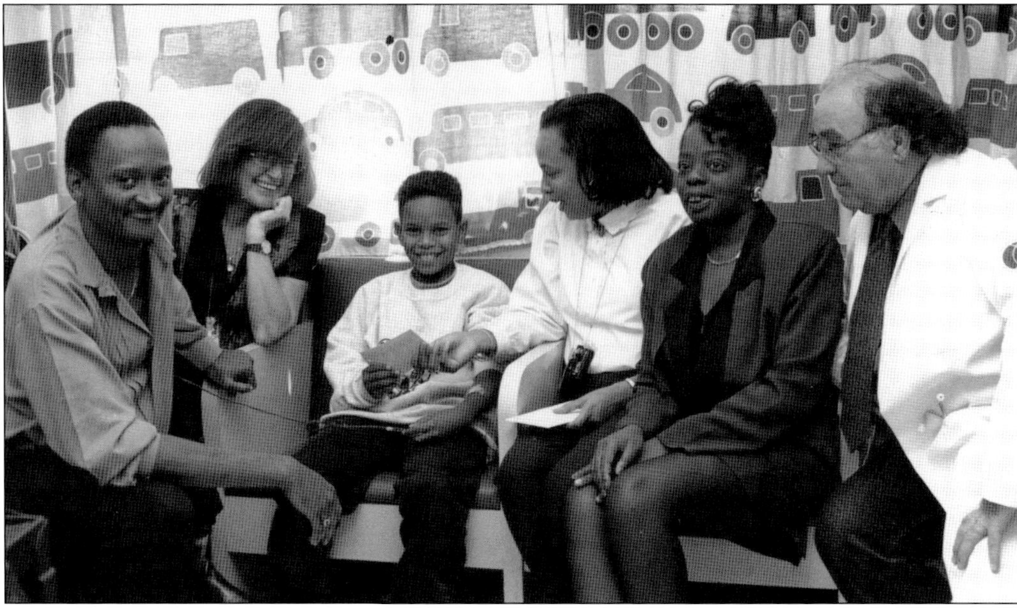

Joan Santos of the Bronx (center) holds a Toys R Us gift certificate for completing a rigorous outpatient treatment regimen for sickle cell anemia at Babies Hospital in 1993. Dr. Sergio Piomelli, director of the hospital's division of hematology-oncology, looks on at right, while Brenda Martin, RN, sickle cell nurse coordinator, at center, hands the reward to Santos. (Photograph by Joan Penn.)

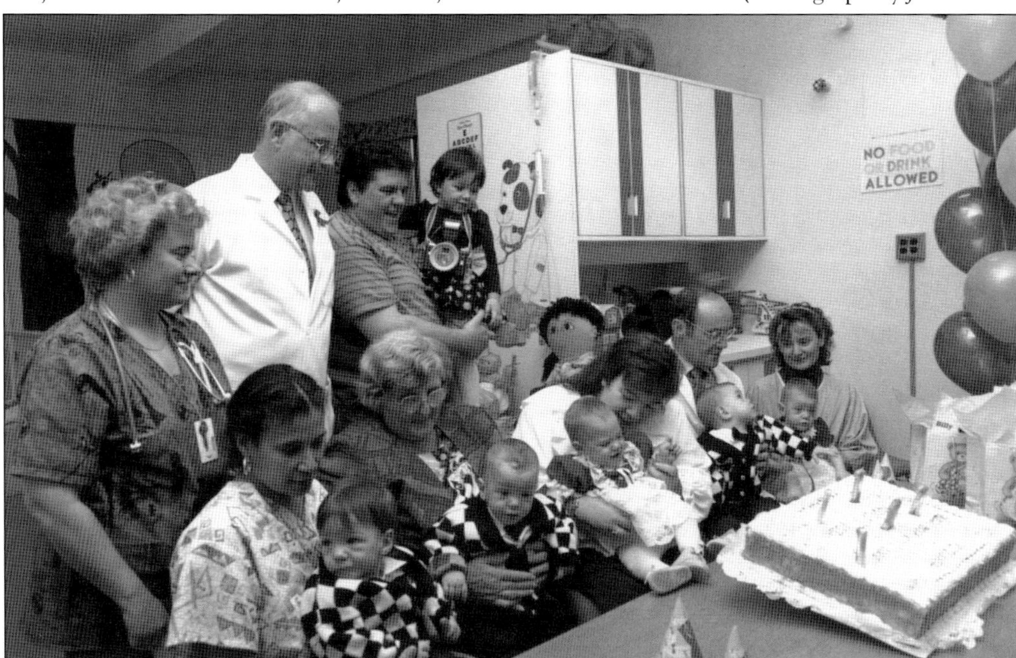

Surrounded by family and the medical team members that cared for them, the Kakkavis quintuplets—Anna, Jimmy, Billy, George, and Aphrodite—celebrate their first birthday at Babies Hospital in the fall of 1993. Standing in the second row, from left to right, are Wendy Cambria, RN, Dr. Harold E. Fox, and father John Kakkavis. Seated in the first row are Carol Robinson, RN, at far left and Drs. Karl Schulze and Helen Towers at far right. (Photograph by Joan Penn.)

Sonia Lagares, RN, explains an immunization record to Audrey Frias in 1995. Frias had brought her infant son to one of Babies Hospital's public school–based clinics for his childhood vaccinations. The clinics helped expand immunization among the children of the hospital's neighborhood of Washington Heights and provided vaccinations free of charge on a walk-in basis for children two and under. (Photograph by Marie Wallace.)

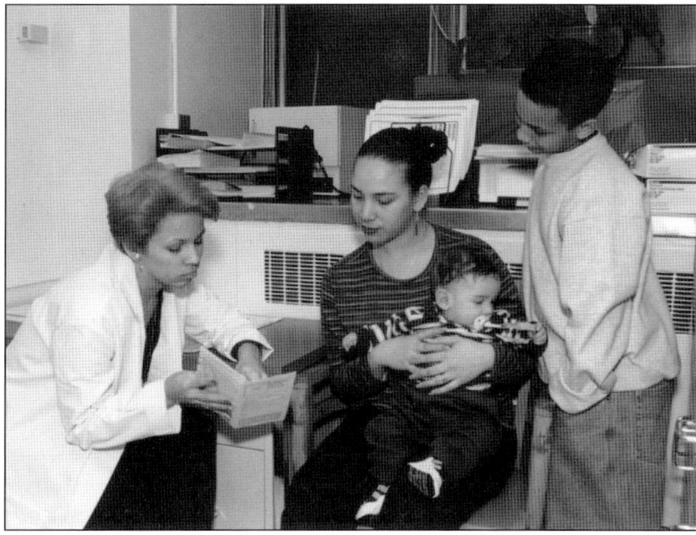

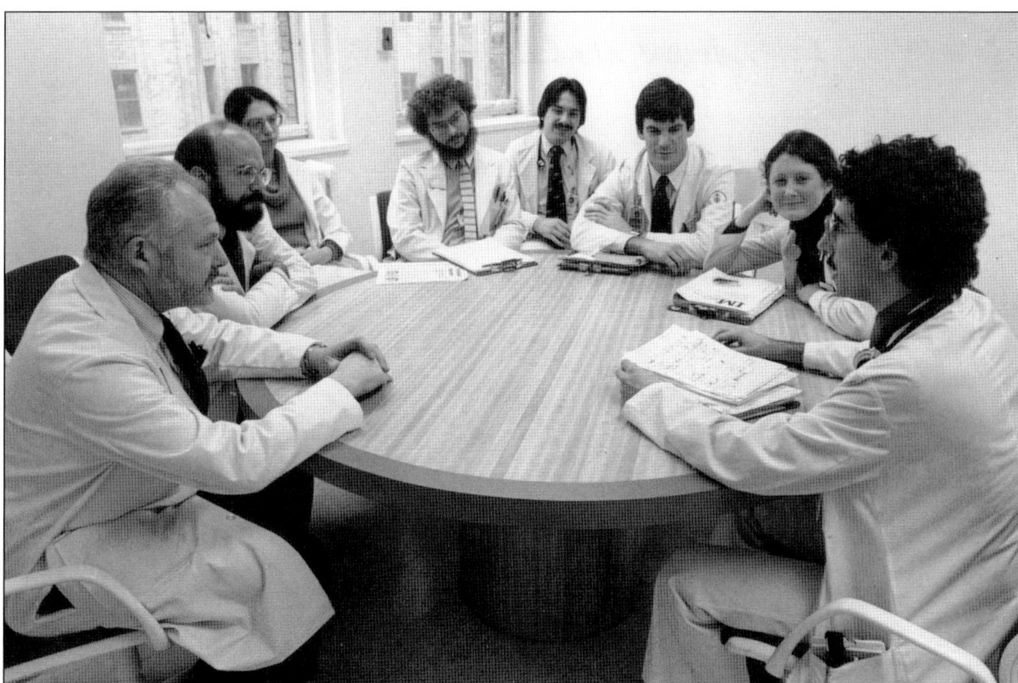

Department chairman Dr. Michael Katz (far left) and Dr. Stephen Atwood, director of the division of medical education (second from left), are seen here in conference with interns and residents around 1980. Atwood had been hired in 1978 to head the division, which oversaw the department's interns and residents. It was needed, too: between 1950 and 1979, the number of interns and residents almost doubled, growing from 23 to 44.

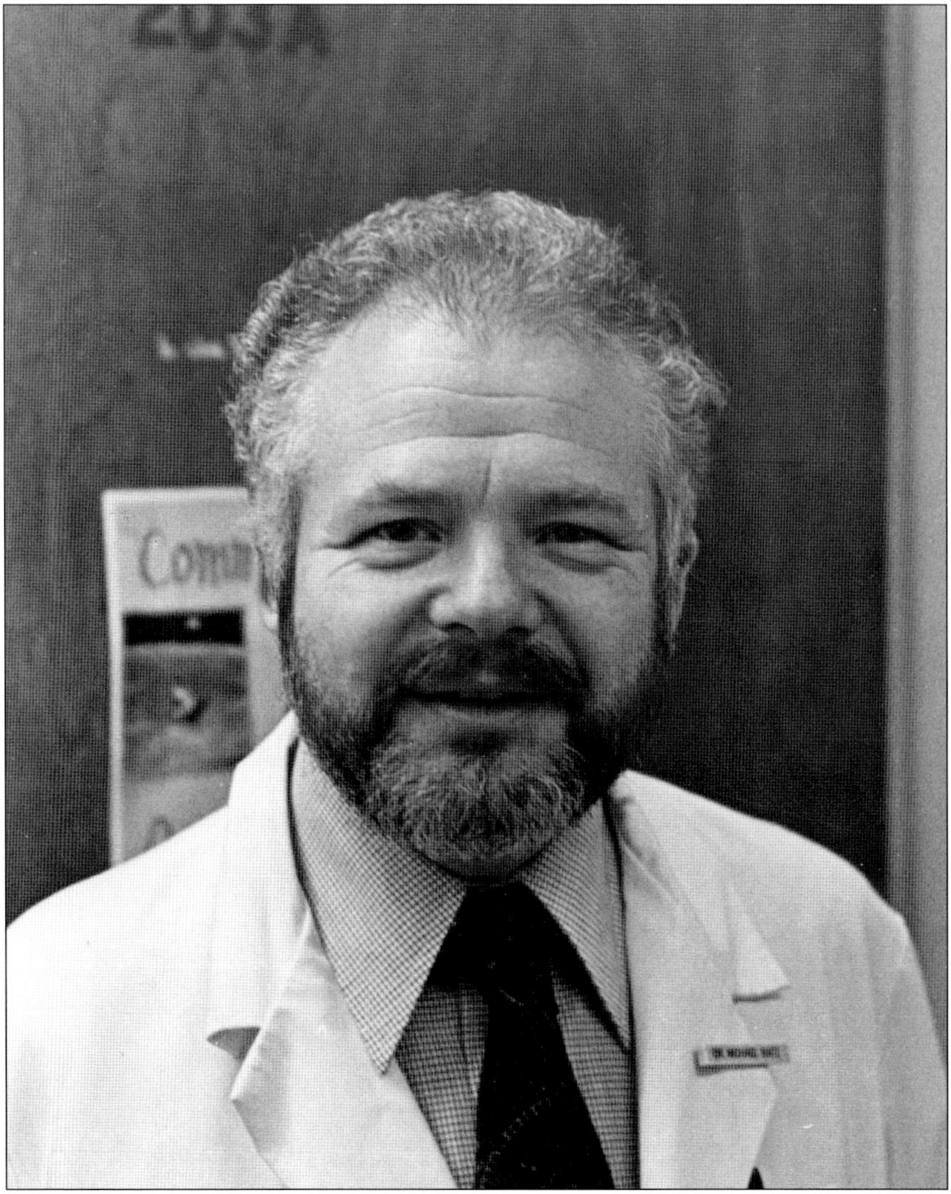

Michael Katz was born in pre–World War II Poland and later immigrated to the United States. He received an artium baccalaureus from the University of Pennsylvania, a master's of science in tropical medicine from Columbia University, and a medical degree from the State University of New York, Downstate Medical Center. He completed a residency at the Babies Hospital and joined the faculty at Columbia University. He was appointed professor of public health and head of the division of tropical medicine in the School of Public Health at Columbia in 1970. Two years later, he became Reuben S. Carpentier Professor, director of pediatrics, and the pediatrician-in-chief at Babies Hospital, positions he held until 1992. He later served as the vice president for research at the March of Dimes Birth Defects Foundation and as a consultant to the World Health Organization. He is a fellow and a 50-year life member of the American Society for the Advancement of Science, a fellow of the Infectious Disease Society of America, and a member of the National Academy of Medicine.

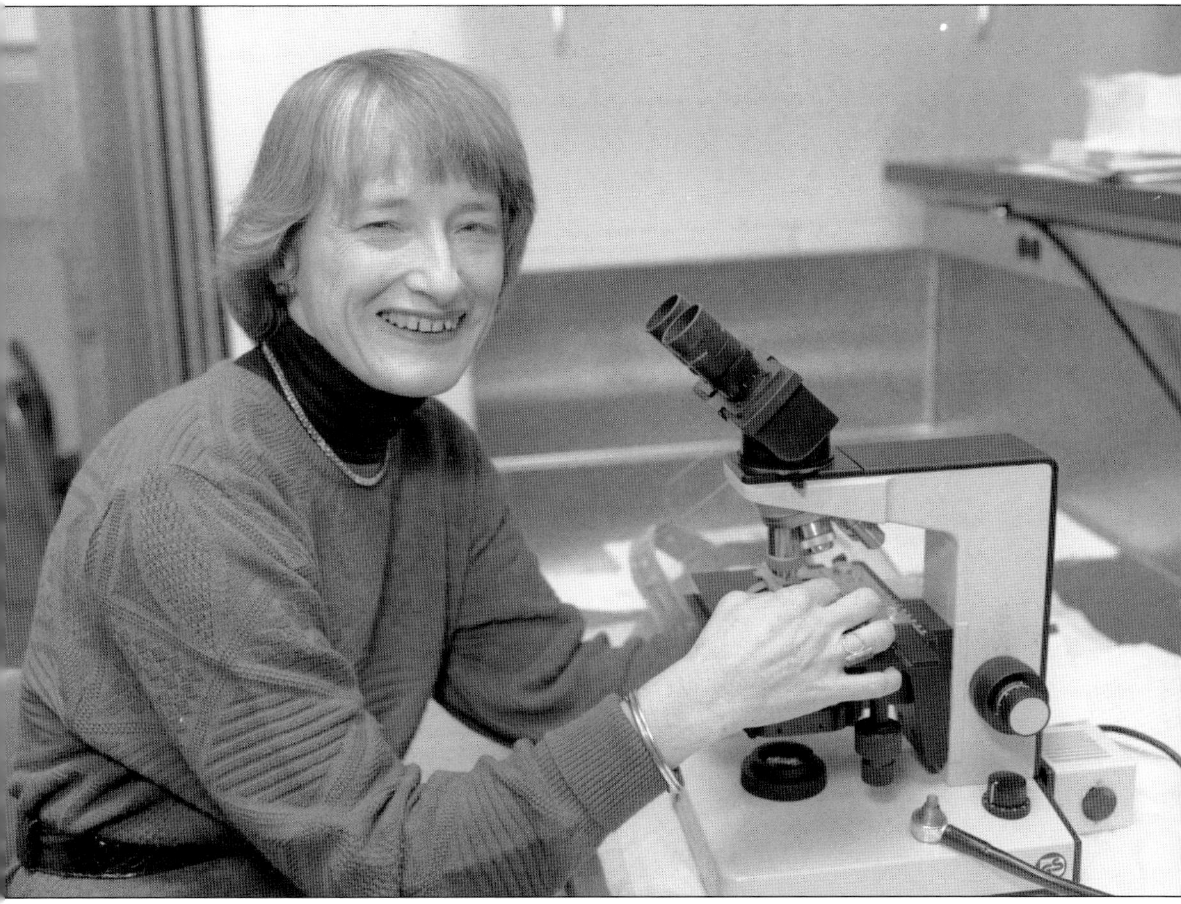

A graduate of Smith College and Cornell University Medical College, Dr. Anne Gershon joined the faculty at the Babies Hospital, Columbia University, as director of pediatric infectious diseases in 1986. She led the original studies for varicella vaccine development in the United States. Originally focused on children with leukemia who were immunocompromised and particularly susceptible to the virus, Dr. Gershon's studies showed that the vaccine was both effective and safe and protected children who were in remission with leukemia from varicella. This research paved the way for the vaccination of varicella in healthy children. In 1995, the vaccine was licensed for use in the United States and dramatically reduced the number of chickenpox cases and varicella-related deaths. In 2013, Dr. Gershon received the Albert B. Sabin Gold Medal from the Sabin Vaccine Institute for her groundbreaking research and leadership. (Photograph by Virgil Sweeden.)

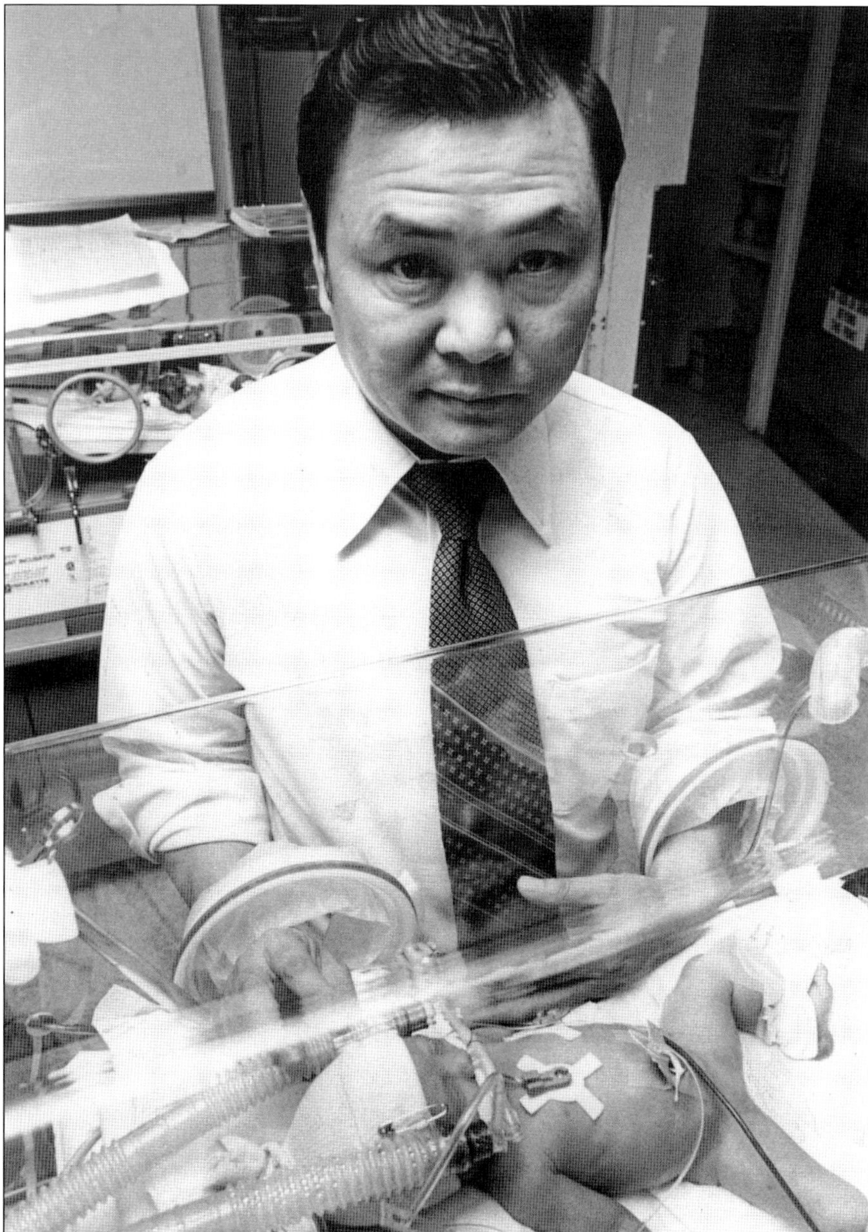

Dr. Jen-Tien Wung, a Taiwanese American neonatologist, graduated from Taipei Medical College and completed residencies in obstetrics-gynecology and anesthesiology at Bronx-Lebanon Hospital Center and the Columbia-Presbyterian Medical Center in New York City in 1971. He then completed a combined fellowship in pediatrics and neonatal intensive care medicine at Babies Hospital and joined the faculty in 1974. Working with colleagues Drs. L. Stanley James and John Driscoll, he pioneered and developed the use of noninvasive nasal continuous positive airway pressure (CPAP), a technique that reduced the need for invasive mechanical ventilation and improved survival rates for premature, extremely low-birth-weight infants. The system, called Bubble CPAP, used short nasal prongs as ventilatory support and revolutionized newborn care. Wung has authored at least 50 published articles and books.

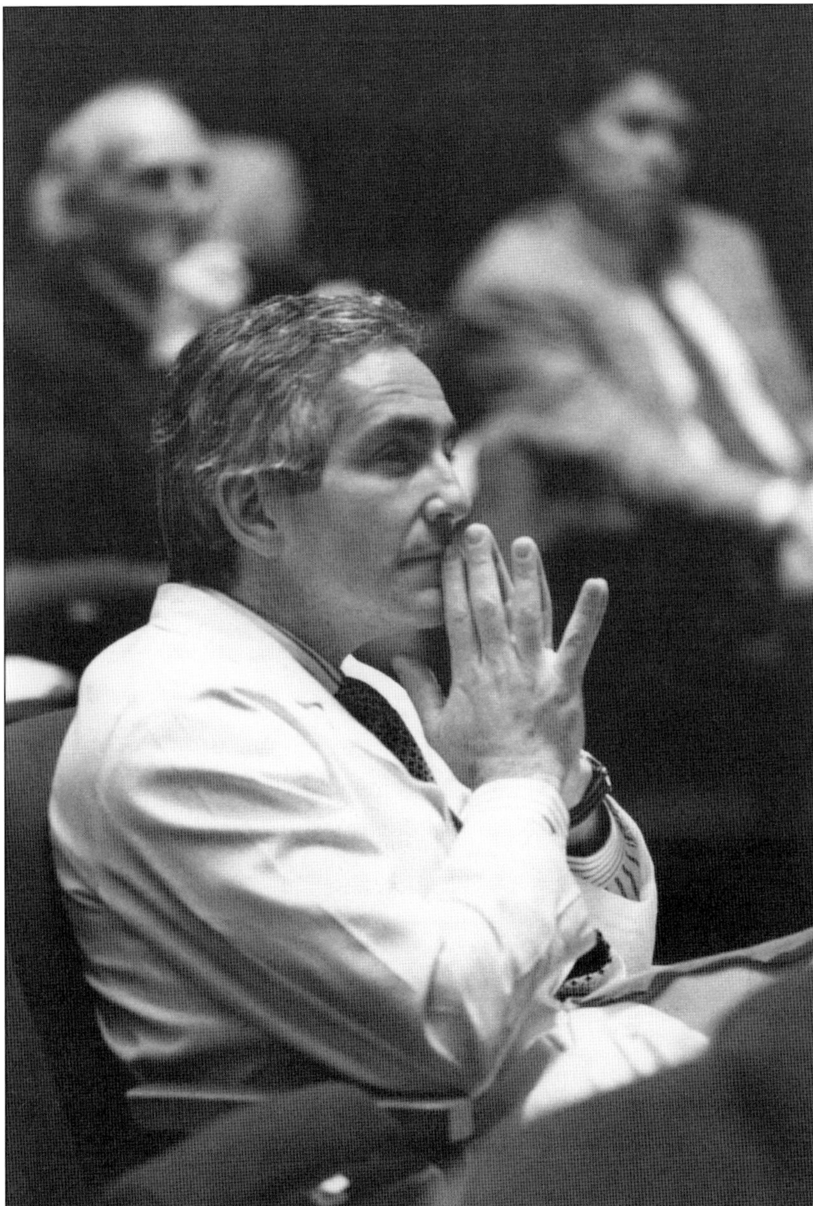

Eric Rose, MD, is a native New Yorker who received his undergraduate degree from Columbia University and his medical degree from Columbia's College of Physicians and Surgeons. He completed his surgical residency and training in cardiothoracic surgery at the Columbia-Presbyterian Medical Center. During his career at Columbia, Dr. Rose held numerous positions, including chair of the department of surgery, director of the clinical perfusion service and of the surgical cardiac intensive care unit, chief of the cardiothoracic surgical service, the Morris and Rose Milstein Professor of Surgery, and associate dean for translational research. He was a pioneer in the use of the implantable left ventricular assist device in patients with severe heart failure. In 1984, Dr. Rose and his surgical team performed one of the earliest successful heart transplants in a pediatric patient. Later in his career, Dr. Rose was an entrepreneur and founder of several biotechnology companies.

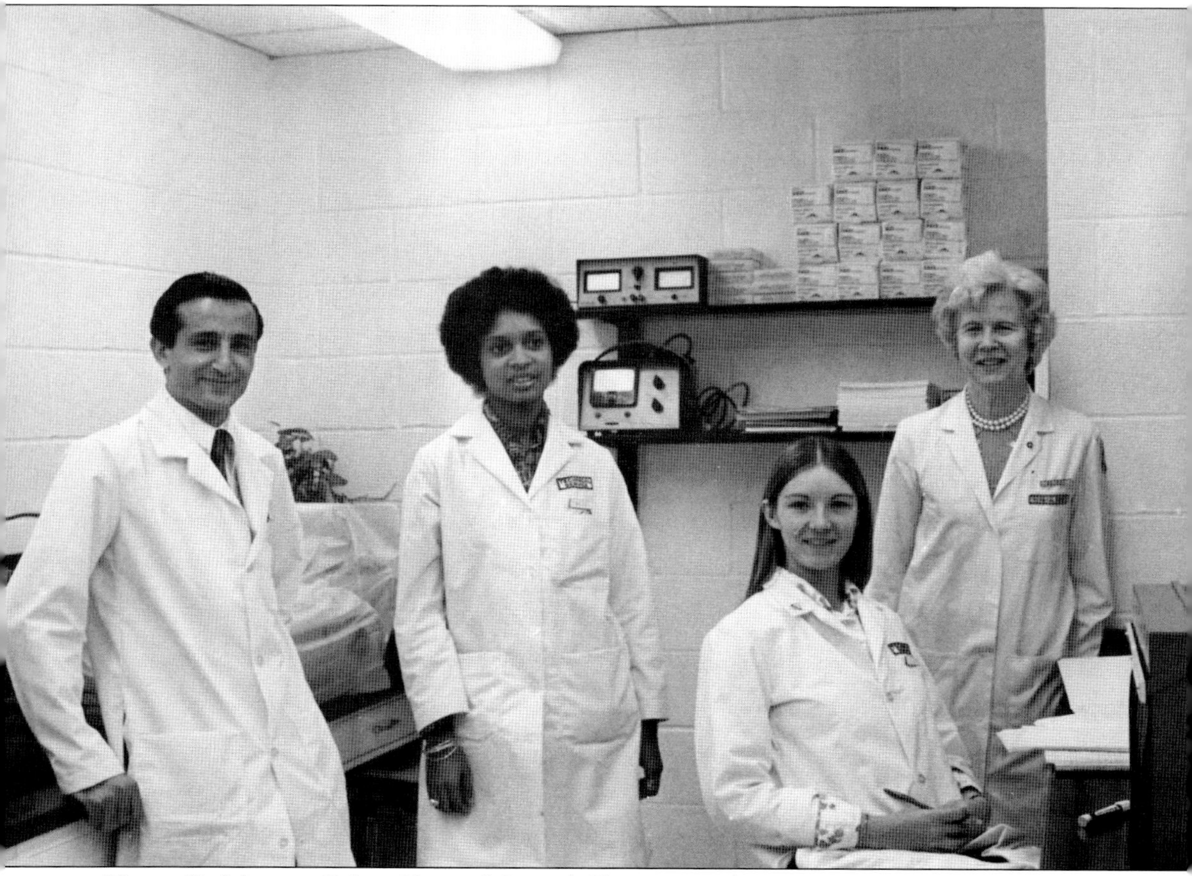

The staff of the new Babies Hospital Special Chemistry Laboratory poses for a group portrait to accompany an article on the laboratory that appeared in the November 1974 issue of the medical center newsletter the *Stethoscope*. Located in what was then known as the Babies Hospital's South Building (now the Central Building), the laboratory undertook a wide variety of tests for the hospital, including those for serum protein electrophoresis, LDH isoenzymes, pheochromocytoma screening, urine electrophoresis, CPK isoenzymes, and electrophoresis, as well as quantification of specific proteins such as immunoglobulins. The unit built on the long history of laboratory testing and research at Babies Hospital. The staff from left to right are Khairy "Ray" Azab, assistant supervisor; Norma Scott, technician; Marina Geipel, technician; and Genevieve C. Corolo, supervisor. (Photograph by Lucy Lazzopina.)

Six

Morgan Stanley Children's Hospital

On January 1, 1998, the NewYork-Presbyterian Hospital was formed by the full asset merger of Columbia-Presbyterian Medical Center and the New York Hospital. However, the two respective Ivy League medical schools, the College of Physician & Surgeons of Columbia University and Weill Cornell School of Medicine, retained their autonomy. In 2000, the investment banking firm Morgan Stanley Dean Witter donated $80 million to build a 21st-century children's hospital on a vacant lot adjacent to the central building of the Babies Hospital on the corner of Broadway and 165th Street in the Washington Heights section of northern Manhattan.

The new 243-bed tower, opened in 2003, provided an improved, modern facility with enhanced and expanded neonatal intensive care and critical care units, a modern 50-bay emergency department, and renovated operating rooms and recovery suites. The new facility provides improved quality of health care to patients and families, enhanced availability of clinical services, and the opportunity to continue the tradition of discovery and innovation.

In recognition of the contribution of Morgan Stanley and its employees, the name of the hospital was changed from the Babies Hospital to the Morgan Stanley Children's Hospital of NewYork-Presbyterian Columbia University Irving Medical Center.

Programs of distinction at the former Babies Hospital of New York include general pediatrics, cancer, digestive disorders, heart and heart surgery, neonatal care, neurology and neurosurgery, and respiratory disorders. As Lawrence R. Stanberry, MD, PhD, the former chairman of pediatrics at the College of Physicians and Surgeons, said: "The focus . . . has not changed in 120 years. We are here to make a difference in the lives of children."

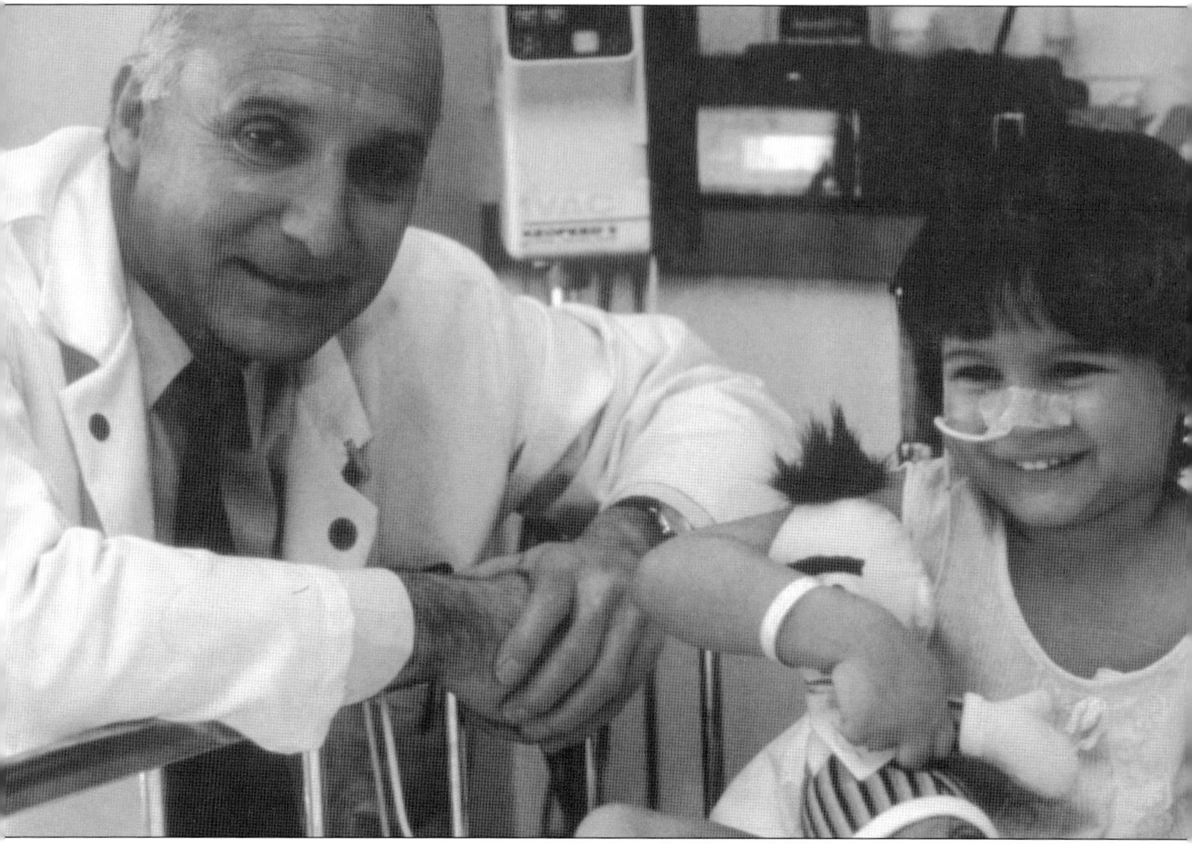

R. Peter Altman, MD, a native New Yorker, attended Colgate University and received his medical degree from the New York Medical College. He served his internship at the Mount Sinai Hospital in New York and trained in general surgery at the Tufts–New England Medical Center and in pediatric surgery at the Children's Hospital National Medical Center in Washington, DC. He joined the Babies Hospital faculty in 1980 as the director of pediatric surgery and surgeon-in-chief. Throughout his career, Dr. Altman was committed to improving and advancing the surgical care of infants and children. His scientific interests centered on hepatobiliary diseases, pediatric surgical oncology, and the development of a staging system for spina bifida and meningomyelocele. Dr. Altman held numerous leadership positions in American surgery. He served as a member of the Residency Review Committee for Surgery and was the president of the American Pediatric Surgical Association. Dr. Altman was a consummate surgeon and educator, training a generation of pediatric surgeons.

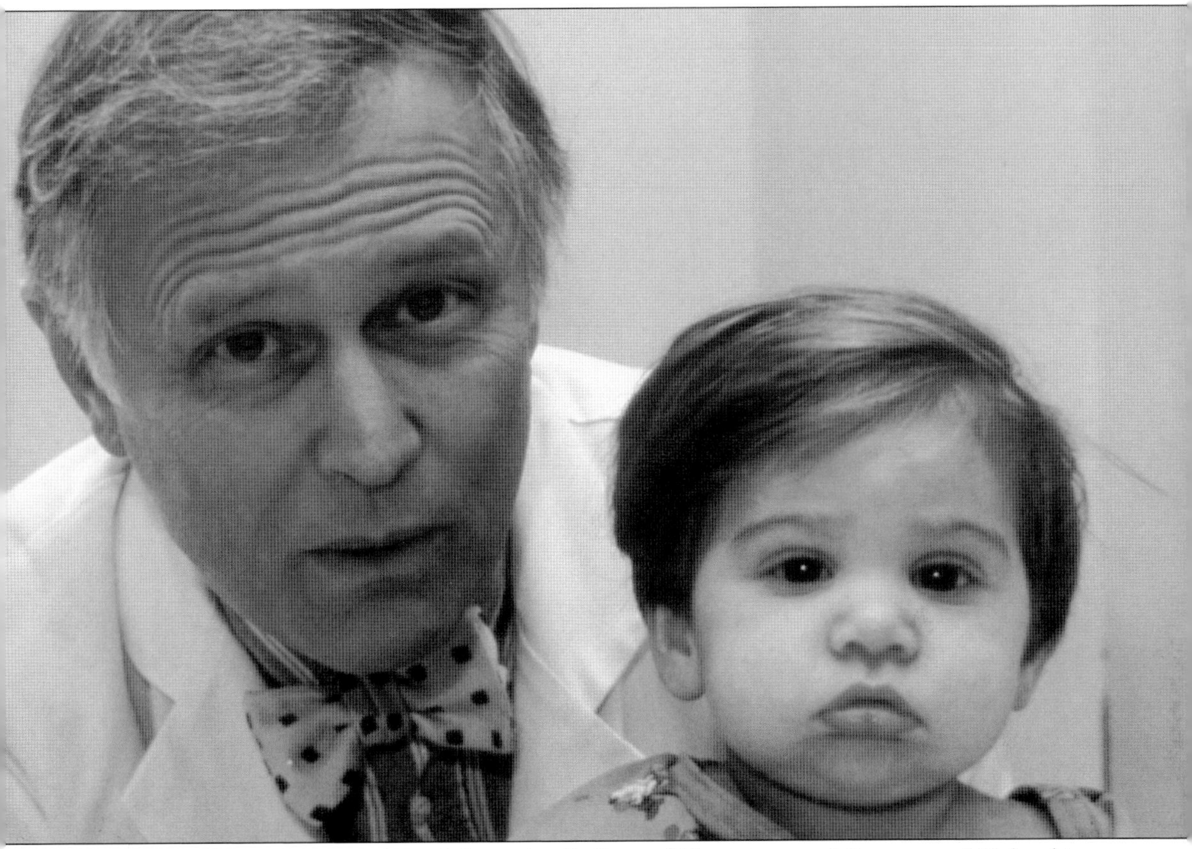

John N. Schullinger, MD, graduated from the College of Physicians and Surgeons of Columbia University in 1955. He completed his surgical training and a subspecialty fellowship in pediatric surgery at Columbia-Presbyterian before joining the full-time faculty. Schullinger trained generations of pediatric surgeons to hone their skills in the treatment of the youngest and most vulnerable. He worked for many years on behalf of the Children of China Pediatrics Foundation to treat surgically correctable deformities of Chinese orphans and to train young Chinese surgeons to do the same. He had particular expertise in neonatal surgery and the care of pediatric cancer and gastroesophageal reflux. He received the 1989 P&S Alumni Medal for meritorious service to the medical school and its alumni, the 1992 Gold Medal for conspicuous service to Columbia University and its alumni, the 1994 Practitioner of the Year Award of the Columbia-Presbyterian Medical Center, the 1995 Arnold P. Gold Award, and the 2003 P&S Alumni Gold Medal for excellence in clinical medicine.

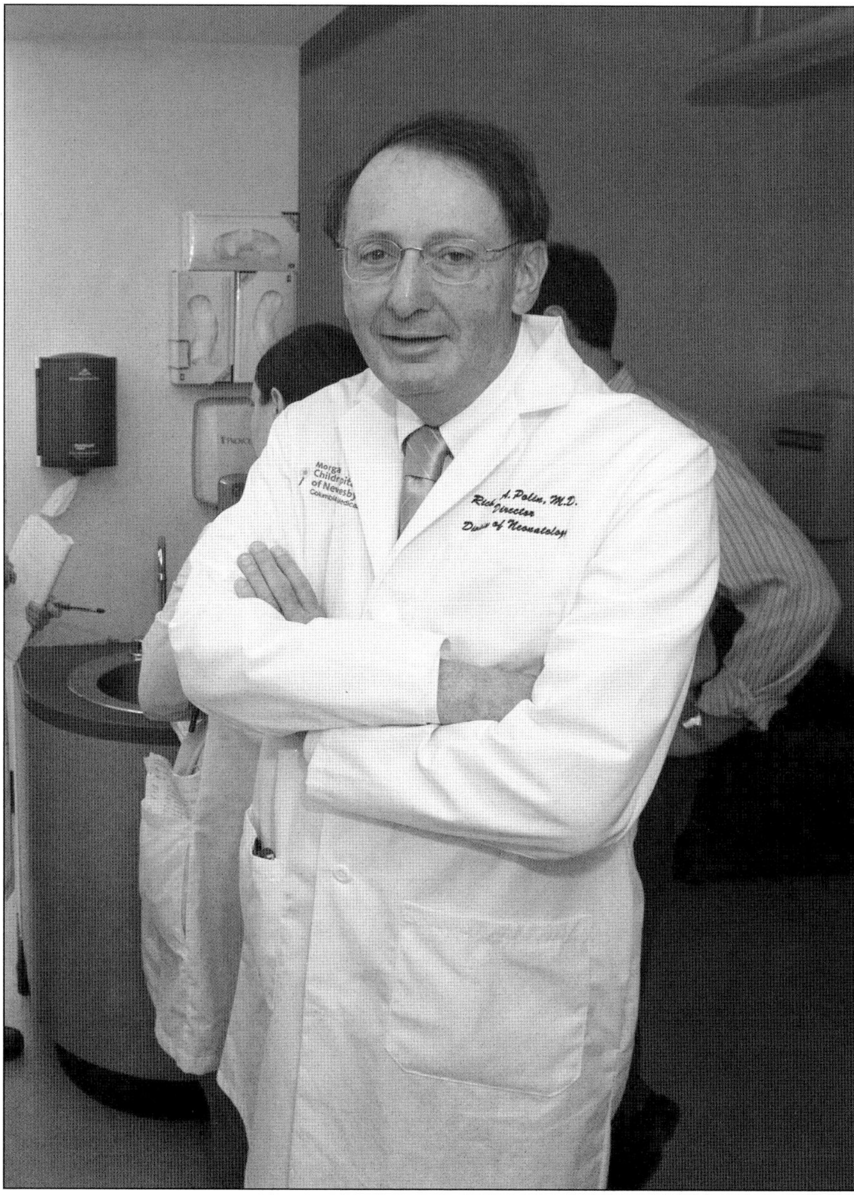

Dr. Richard A. Polin is the William T. Speck Professor of Pediatrics at Columbia University, Vagelos College of Physicians and Surgeons, and former director of the division of neonatology at the Babies Hospital from 1998 to 2019. He earned bachelor of arts and medical degrees from Temple University and completed a pediatric internship and residency at Children's Memorial Hospital in Chicago as well as a pediatric residency and neonatology fellowship at Babies Hospital. Prior to his return to the Babies Hospital in 1998 as the director of neonatology, he was a member of the faculty at the Children's Hospital of Philadelphia. In 2005, he received the Physician of the Year Award both from Columbia University Medical Center and the Morgan Stanley Children's Hospital division of nursing. In the spring of 2006, Dr. Polin received the National Neonatal Education Award from the AAP's Section on Perinatal Pediatrics. Dr. Polin has published over 200 original papers and 20 books, including *Fetal and Neonatal Physiology*, *Workbook in Practical Neonatology*, *Pediatric Secrets*, *Fetal and Neonatal Secrets*, and *Current Pediatric Therapy*.

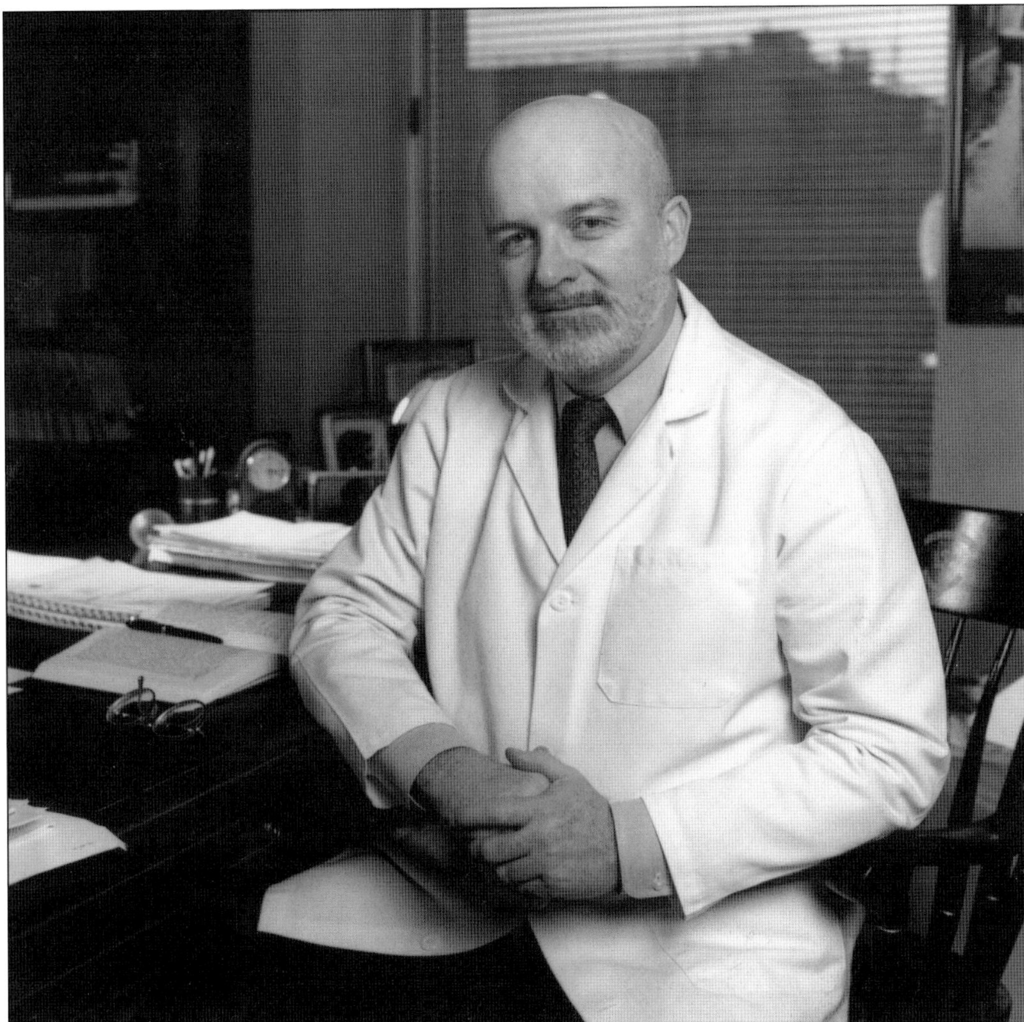

A graduate of Rutgers University and the Wake Forest University School of Medicine, Dr. William Speck's postdoctoral training included a fellowship in infectious disease at the College of Physicians and Surgeons of Columbia University. This led to a joint appointment in the departments of pediatrics and microbiology. He departed Columbia for Case Western Reserve University School of Medicine and the Rainbow Babies and Children's Hospital, where he served as chairman of the department of pediatrics for 10 years. In 1992, Dr. Speck returned to the Columbia-Presbyterian Medical Center as chief executive officer and president and was responsible for its merger with New York Hospital on December 31, 1997. He became the first president of the new entity, the New York-Presbyterian Hospital, the largest academic medical center in the country. Today, Dr. Speck is an emeritus professor of clinical pediatrics at the College of Physicians and Surgeons of Columbia University, where he is involved in house officer education and serves on its institutional review board. He is copresident of City Meals on Wheels, a major nonprofit social service organization in New York City.

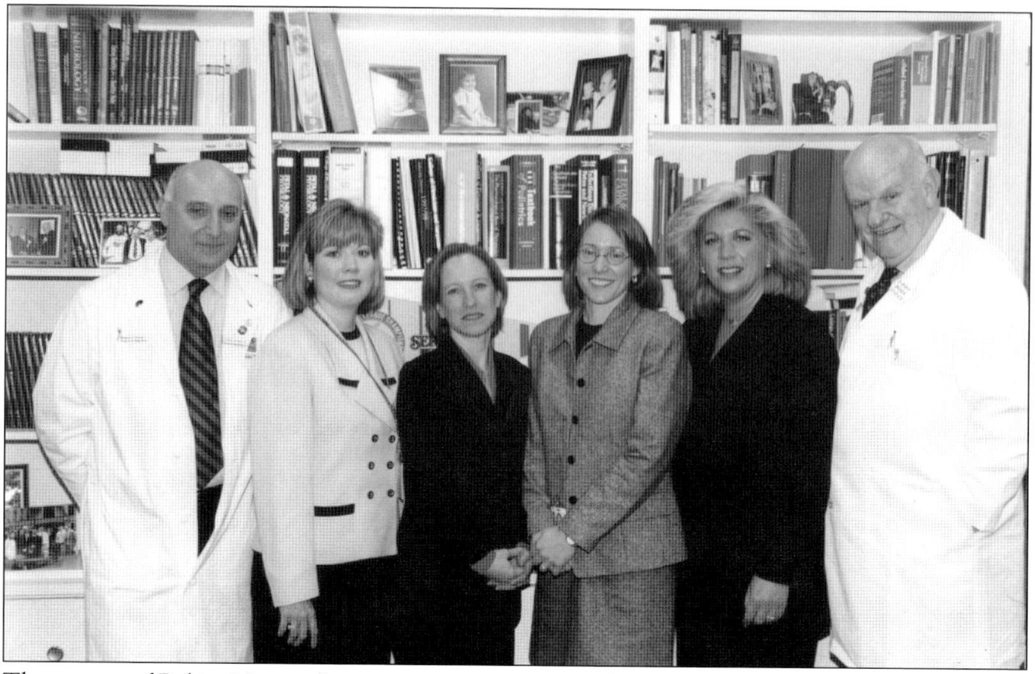

The merger of Babies Hospital's parent organization, Presbyterian Hospital, with crosstown rival New York Hospital in late 1997 resulted in the leadership team seen here in November 1998. From left to right are R. Peter Altman, surgeon-in-chief; Theresa Larivee, director of operations; Andrea Bembry, RN, vice president for patient care services; Gigi Madore, director of pediatric outreach, Cynthia Sparer, senior vice president; and John Driscoll, director and physician-in-chief. (Photograph by Marie Wallace.)

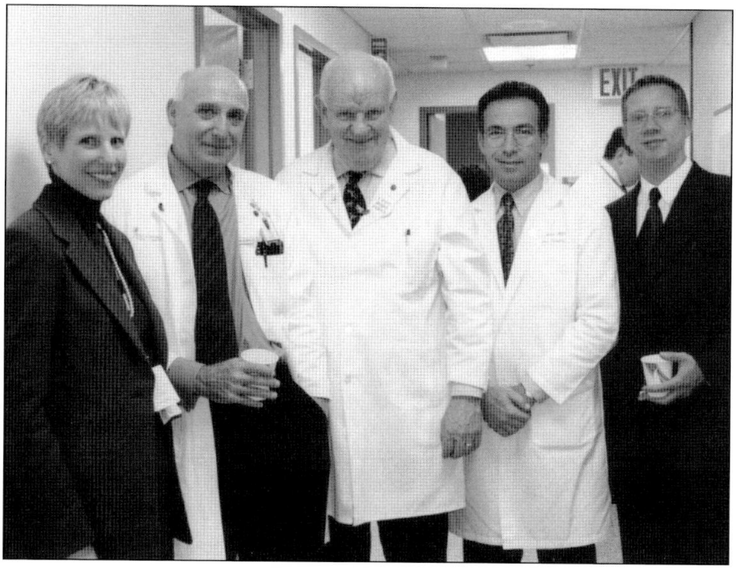

The opening of a newly renovated and enlarged pediatric emergency room was cause for celebration in November 1999. Seen here at the ribbon-cutting ceremony are, from left to right, unidentified; Dr. R. Peter Altman, director of pediatric surgery, Babies Hospital; Dr. John M. Driscoll, director and department chairman; Steven Stylianos, pediatric surgeon; and unidentified.

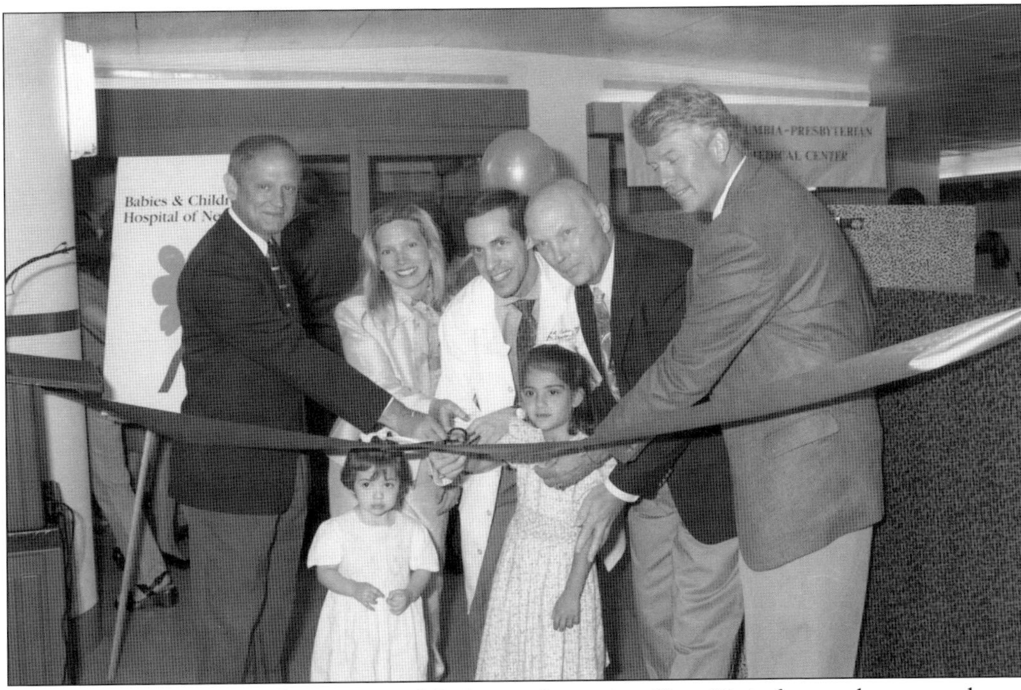

The newly renovated Babies Hospital Pediatric Intensive Care Unit featured a space theme, so who better to inaugurate it than astronauts? Seen here at the June 1998 ribbon-cutting are astronauts Norman Thagard (left), Story Musgrave (MD, Columbia, 1964, second from right), and Byron Lichtenberg (right). Dr. Howard Zucker, director of the Pediatric Intensive Care Unit, is at the center, while nurse unit manager Judi Peacock, RN, is second from left. In front, two former patients, Gabriella Acevedo (left) and Katya Johns (right), assist. The new PICU expanded capacity from 13 to 27 beds and included larger patient rooms, a family lounge, and a quiet room. The reception area (below) featured a photomural of children reaching for the skies. (Above, photograph by Charles E. Manley; below, photograph by Colin McRae.)

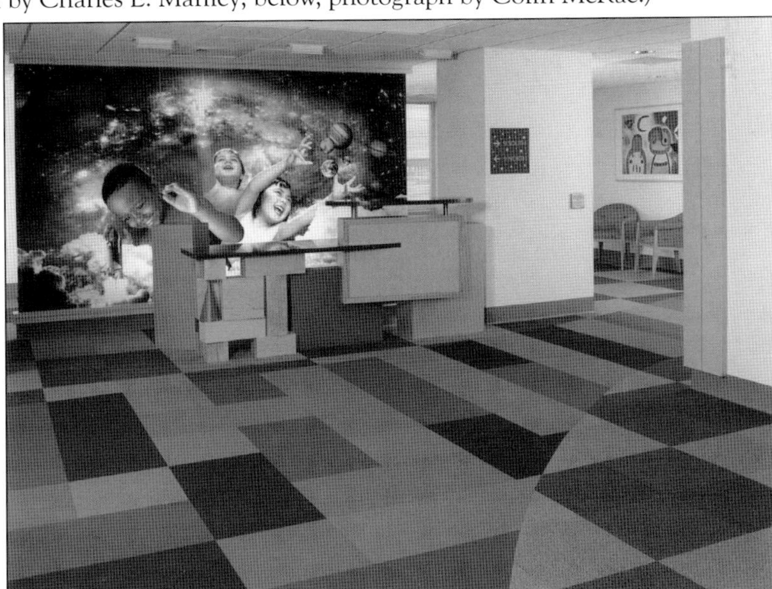

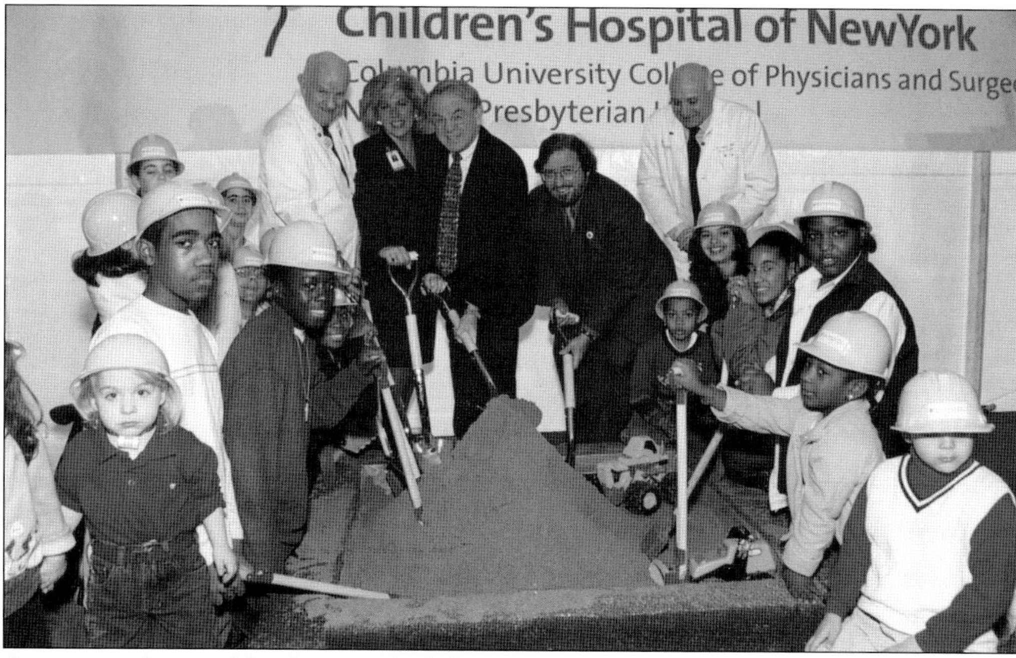

A ceremonial ground breaking marked the construction of a new hospital building, Morgan Stanley Children's Hospital, on November 16, 2000. A phalanx of dignitaries participated, including, from left to right, John C. Driscoll, chairman, department of pediatrics and director, Babies Hospital; Cynthia N. Sparer, senior vice president, NYPH; Herb Pardes, president and chief executive officer, NYPH; New York City councilman Stanley Michels; and R. Peter Altman, director, pediatric surgery. (Photograph by Marie Wallace.)

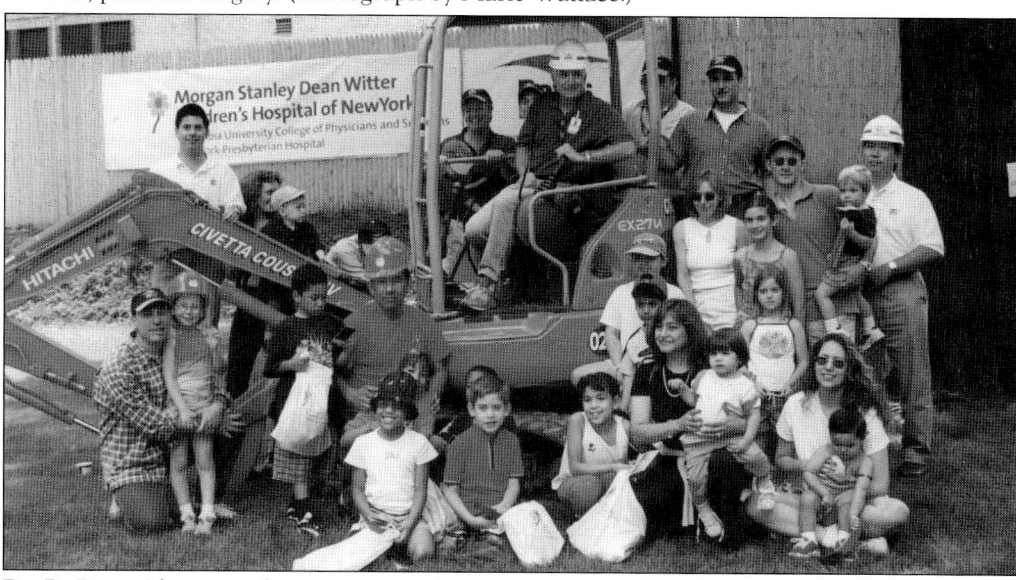

Dr. R. Peter Altman and patients visit the construction site of the Morgan Stanley Children's Hospital with a "hole in the ground" tour on June 9, 2001. The investment banking firm Morgan Stanley Dean Witter supported the construction at Broadway and 165th Street. The new tower added 243 beds to the existing Babies Hospital, and the name forever changed to the Morgan Stanley Children's Hospital of New York. (Photograph by Luisa Engel.)

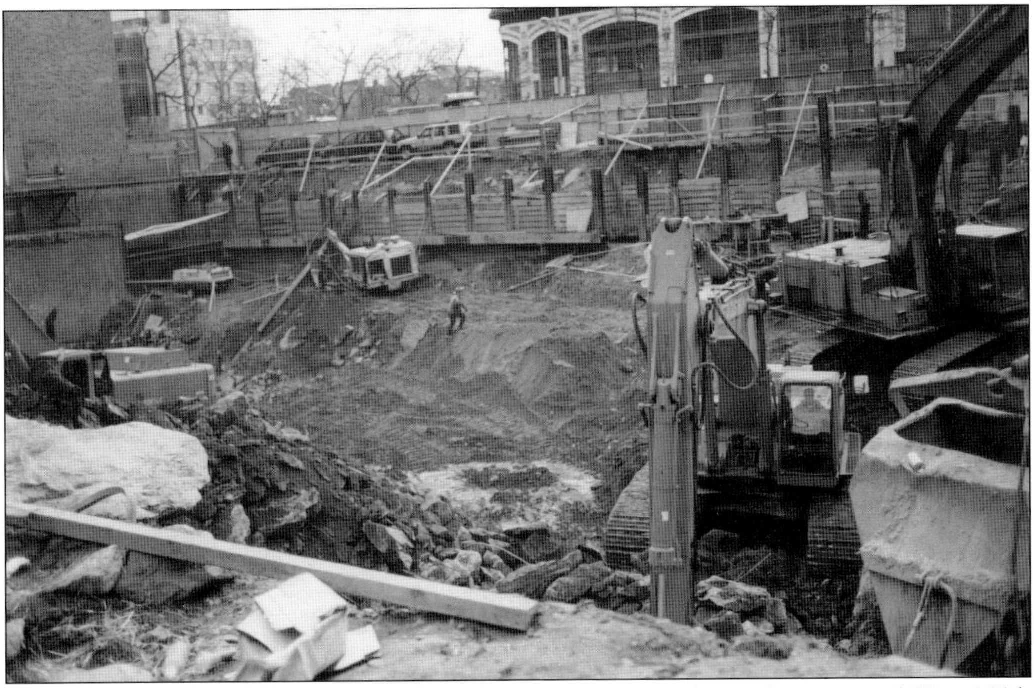

The new Morgan Stanley Children's Hospital was built on a plot at the corner of West 165th Street and Broadway that had been used as a parking lot practically from the time the medical center opened in 1928. On this prominent location rose a 10-story building with 265,000 square feet of space, greatly increasing the scope of the hospital's services. Seen here are construction photographs from the spring of 2001. Above is a view to the east across Broadway with the university's Mary Woodard Lasker Building seen above the construction fence. Below is a view southward across West 165th Street showing the wooden forms for the foundation walls. (Both photographs by Constance H. Halporn.)

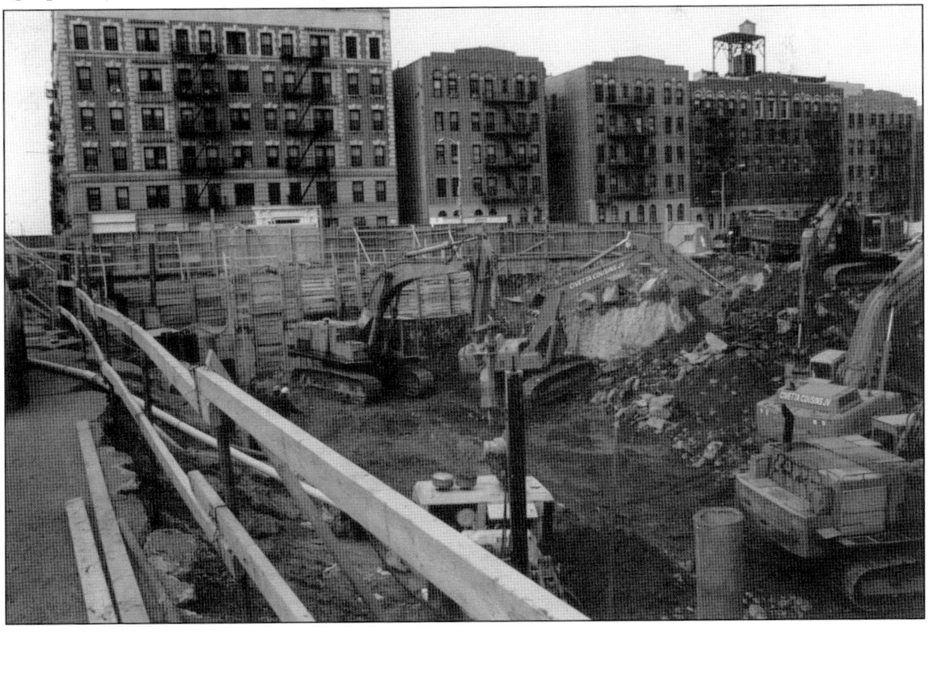

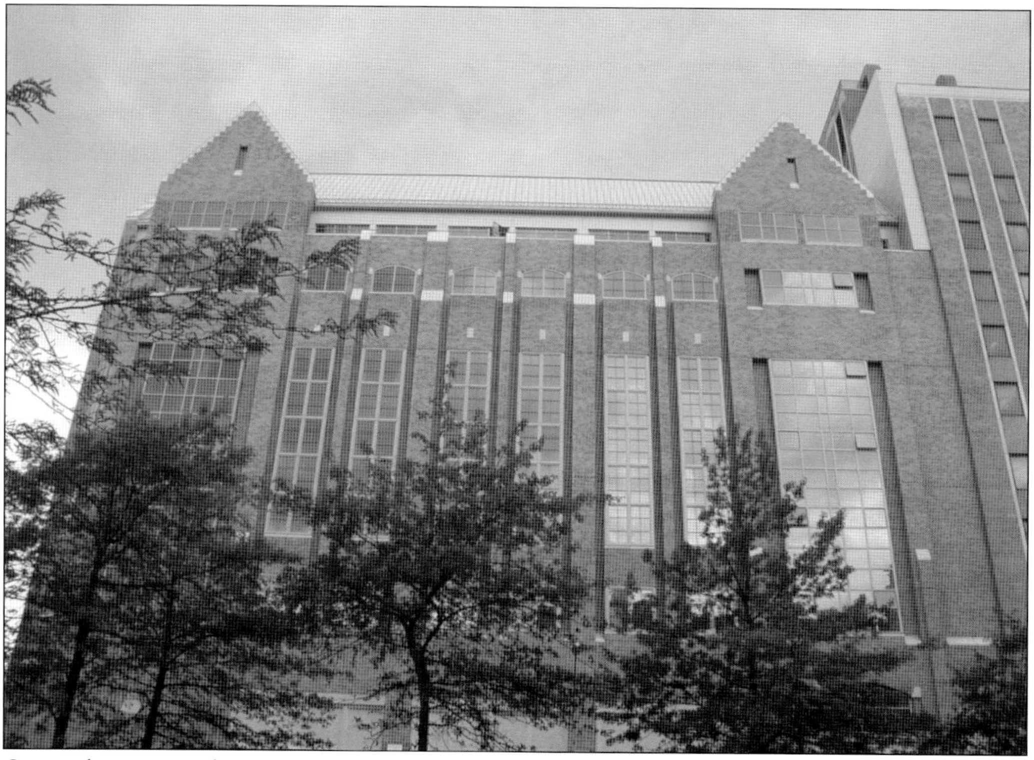

Opened in 2003, the new Morgan Stanley Children's Hospital was designed by the noted architectural firm Davis Brody Bond. Its style, modeled after that of late-19th-century Scottish architect Charles Rennie Mackintosh, was a sharp break from the hospital's earlier architecture. The $55 million needed to complete the building was raised by more than 300 employees of the financial services firm Morgan Stanley. (Photograph by Charles E. Manley.)

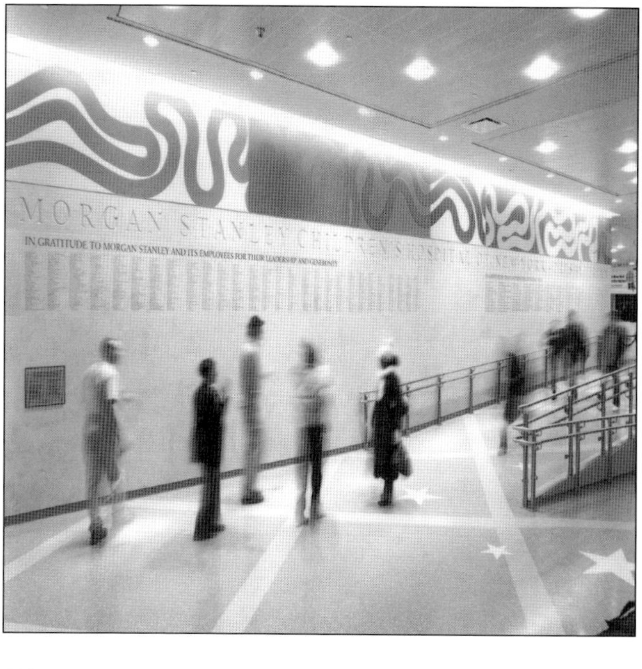
MORGAN STANLEY
IN GRATITUDE TO MORGAN STANLEY AND ITS EMPLOYEES

Among the striking features of the new Morgan Stanley Children's Hospital is its abundance of art. Perhaps the most important work is the vibrant mural by Sol LeWitt that runs along the top of the lobby walls entitled *Wall Drawing No. 1109*, seen here. LeWitt (1928–2007) worked in a wide variety of media and is considered one of the founders of minimalism and conceptual art.

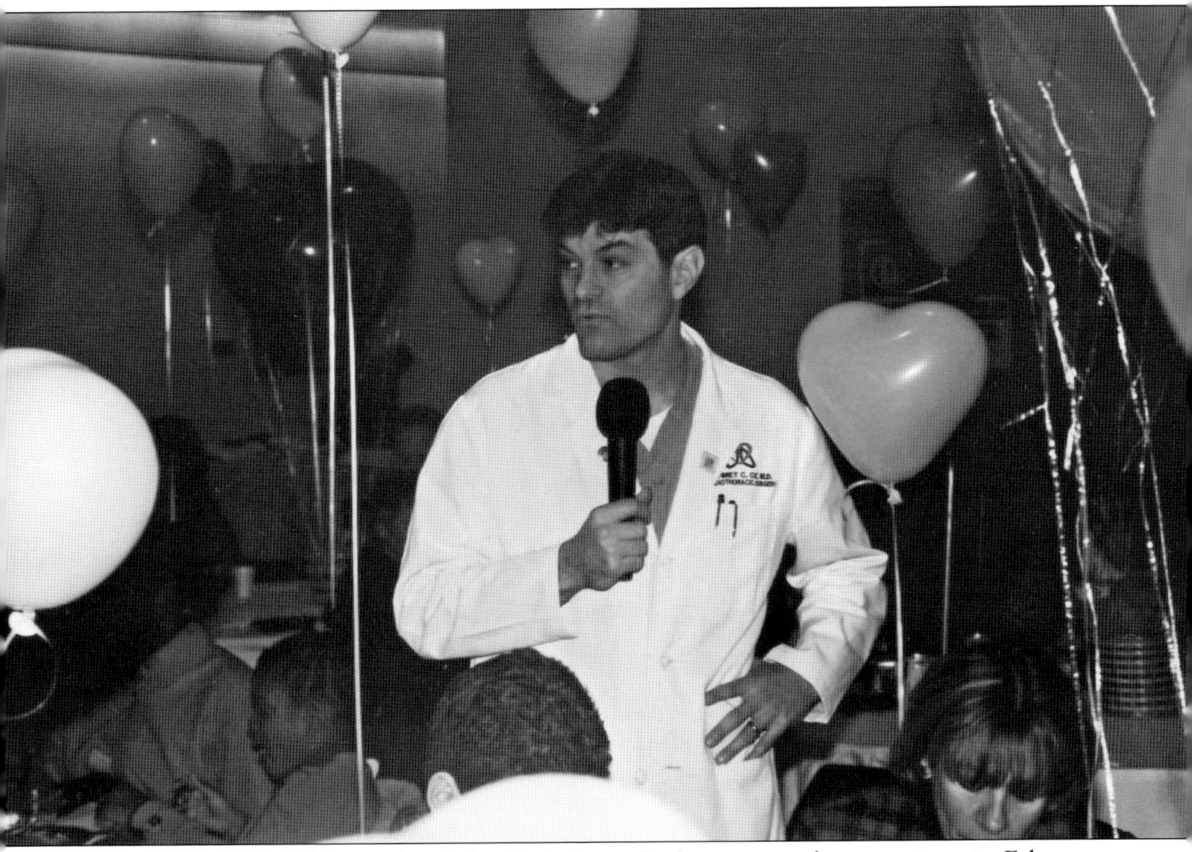

Mehmet Oz, MD, addresses the Gift of Life Party for heart transplant survivors in February 2001. Dr. Oz, a cardiothoracic surgeon at Columbia University Medical Center, received his undergraduate degree from Harvard and medical and master of business administration degrees simultaneously from the University of Pennsylvania. He was a professor of surgery and director of the Cardiovascular Institute and Complementary Medicine Program at Columbia. He developed a technique to use a single suture to close leaks in the mitral valve and was an advocate of a ventricular assist device as an alternative for patients with heart failure. Oprah Winfrey launched his television career, originally with a series on the Discovery Channel, *Second Opinion with Dr. Oz*. He became a frequent guest on *The Oprah Winfrey Show* and, in 2009, began *The Dr. Oz Show*, produced by Harpo Productions and Sony Pictures Television. (Photograph by Brian Dotson.)

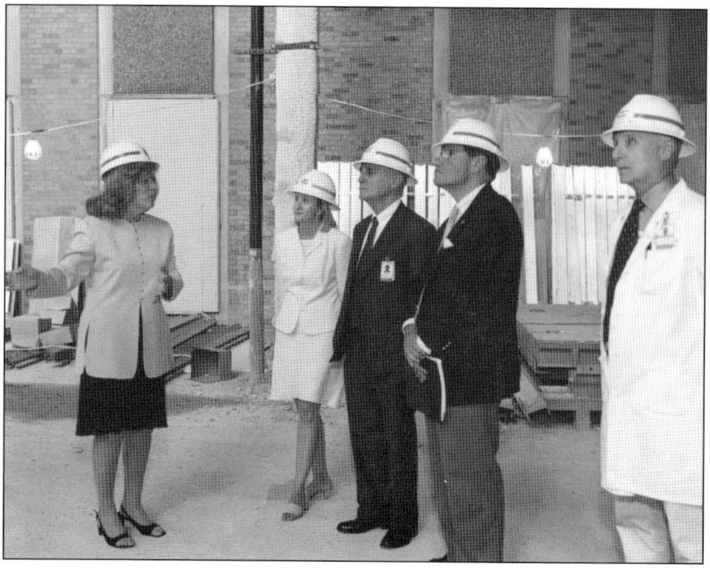

Cynthia Sparer (left), executive director of the Morgan Stanley Children's Hospital of New York, and Dr. R. Peter Altman (right) tour the new construction site on July 24, 2001, with unidentified members of the New York-Presbyterian Hospital board of trustees. The new bed tower was connected internally to the former Babies Hospital North Building, erected in 1929, and the Central Building, constructed in the early 1960s. (Photograph by Eileen Miller.)

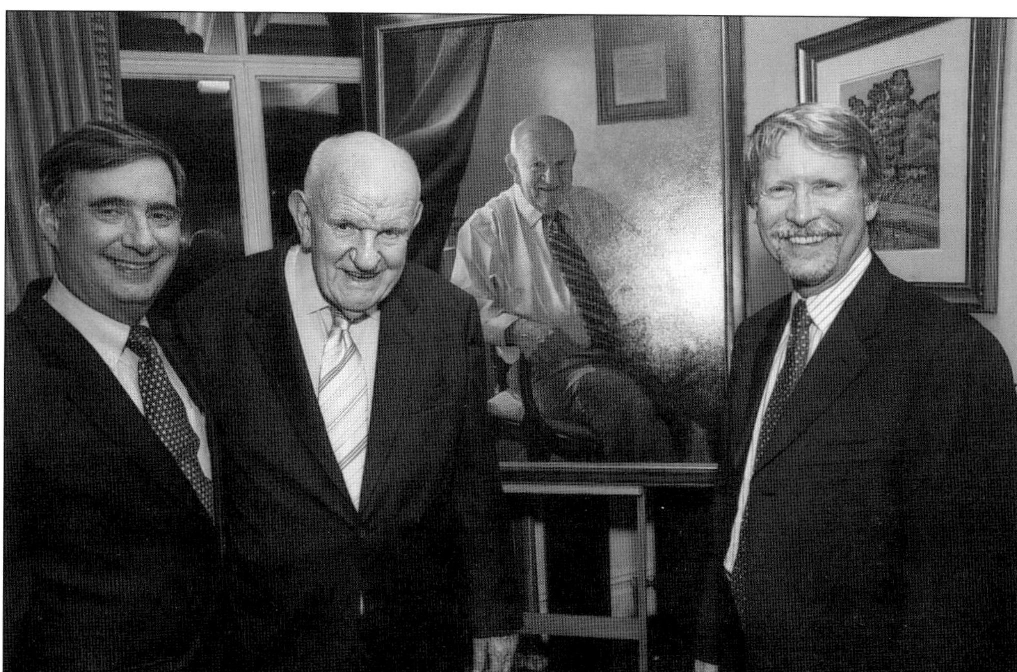

John Driscoll's tenure as director of Morgan Stanley Children's Hospital and chairman of the department of pediatrics was commemorated in March 2011 with the unveiling of his portrait. Standing before it are, from left to right, Dr. Lee Goldman, Columbia University dean and executive vice president for health and biomedical sciences; Driscoll; and his successor as hospital director, Dr. Lawrence R. Stanberry. Painted by artist-physician Christopher French, the portrait was donated by Clare Matschullat.

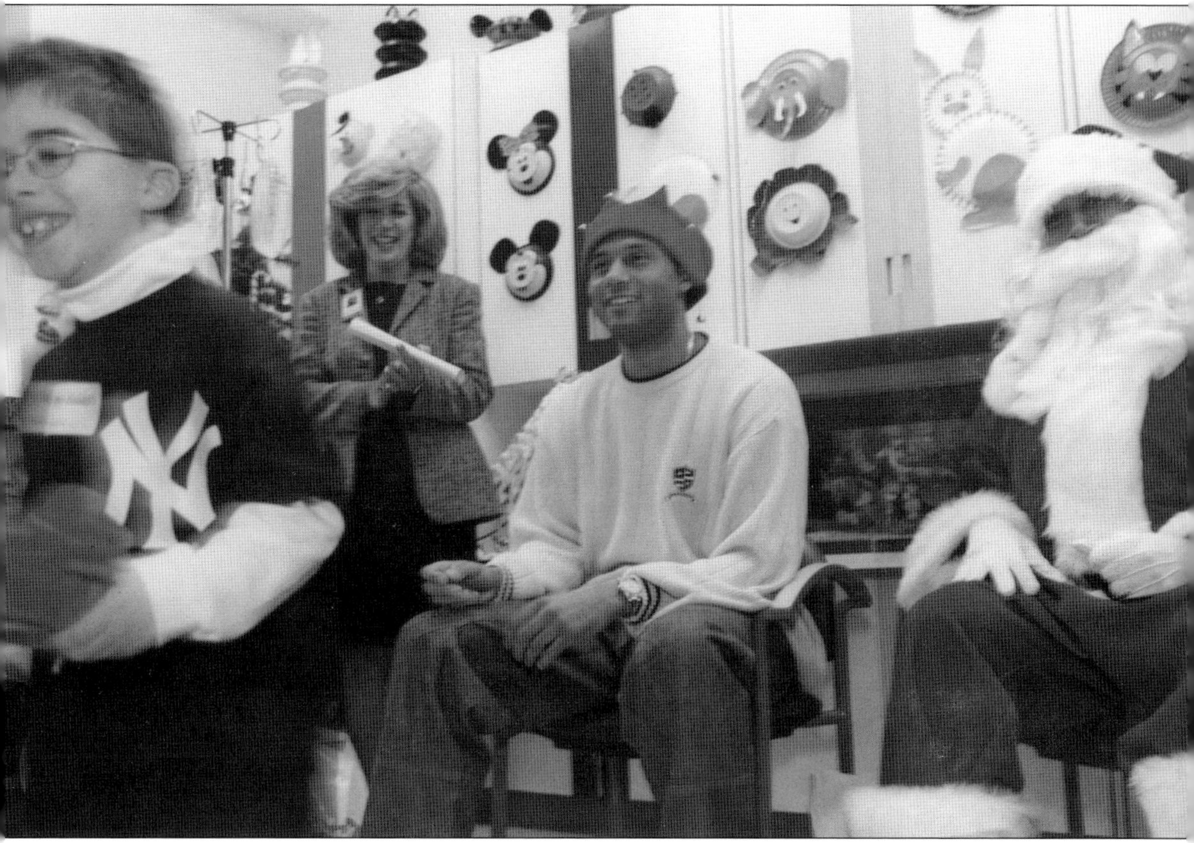

Derek Jeter, famed New York Yankees great, was a frequent visitor to the Morgan Stanley Children's Hospital and became an avid supporter of its mission. In this photograph, he assists Santa Claus to distribute Christmas gifts on December 18, 2001. Cynthia Sparer, executive vice president of the hospital, looks on as a patient, an avid Yankees fan, accepts a gift from his hero. Jeter, born in New Jersey, spent his entire 20-year career in Yankees pinstripes as their starting shortstop. He played on World Series teams, won a Most Valuable Player award in 2000, and has been named to 14 American League All-Star Teams. Jeter was inducted into the Baseball Hall of Fame in Cooperstown, New York, in July 2021. Upon retiring from baseball, he became a businessman and is a part-owner of the Miami Marlins baseball team in Florida. (Photograph by Eileen Miller.)

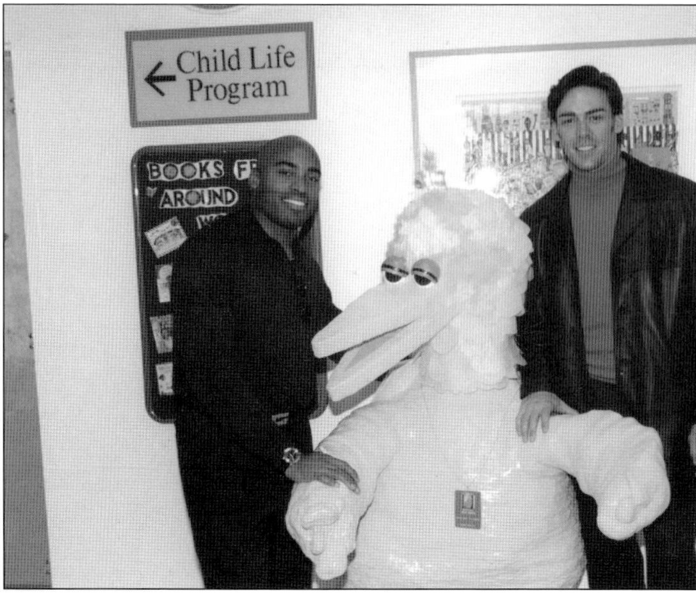

Tiki Barber (left) and Jason Seahorn (right) along with Big Bird visit patients at the Morgan Stanley Children's Hospital on February 13, 2001. New York professional sports heroes are frequent visitors to the hospital. Barber, a New York Football Giants running back, and his teammate Jason Seahorn, a defensive back, enjoyed their time with the patients. (Photograph by Marie Wallace.)

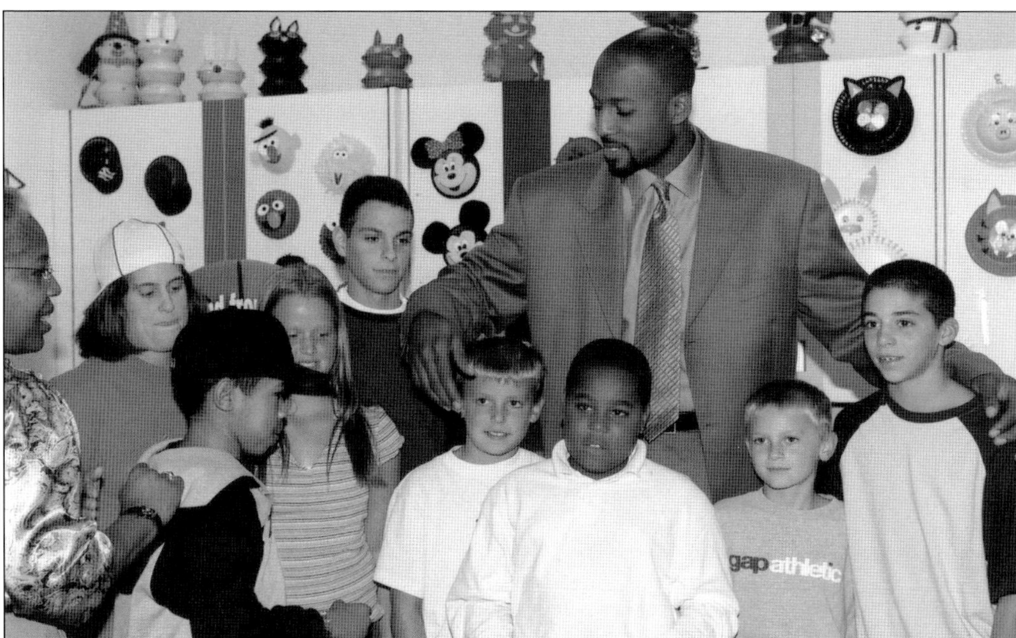

Alonzo Mourning visits patients at the Morgan Stanley Children's Hospital on September 18, 2003. Mourning, a hall-of-fame National Basketball Association megastar, played for the Miami Heat and New Jersey Nets. He established the Alonzo Mourning Charities to aid at-risk children. After being diagnosed with glomerulosclerosis, Mourning created Zo's Fund to raise awareness and funding for research and education in the fight against kidney disease. (Photograph by Janet Charles.)

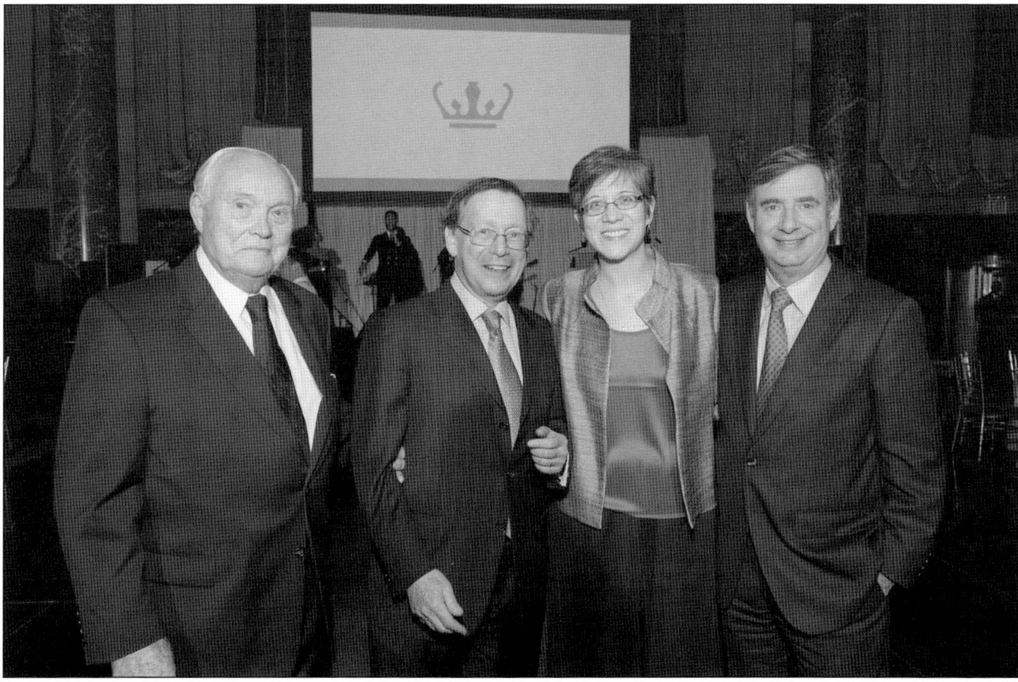

The Babies Heart Fund Cabaret is a major fundraising event for the hospital. Celebrating at the 2013 cabaret are, from left to right, James R. Malm, the first pediatric cardiac surgeon at Babies Hospital; Robert Roskind, founder of the Babies Heart Fund; Julie A. Vincent, chief of pediatric cardiology; and Lee Goldman, dean and executive vice president of the faculties of medicine and biomedical sciences at Columbia University. (Photograph by Michael DeVito.)

The Babies Heart Fund was created by dedicated families to help the division of pediatric cardiology support research and recognize the extraordinary care received by their children. Pictured at the 2014 annual cabaret are, from left to right, Emile Bacha, chief of cardiothoracic surgery; Julie Vincent, director of pediatric cardiology; and Kimara Targoff, recipient of the annual research award. (Photograph by Michael DeVito.)

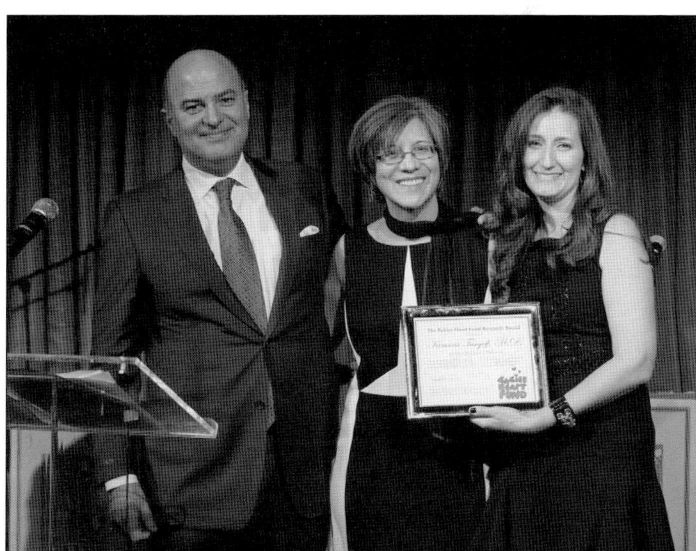

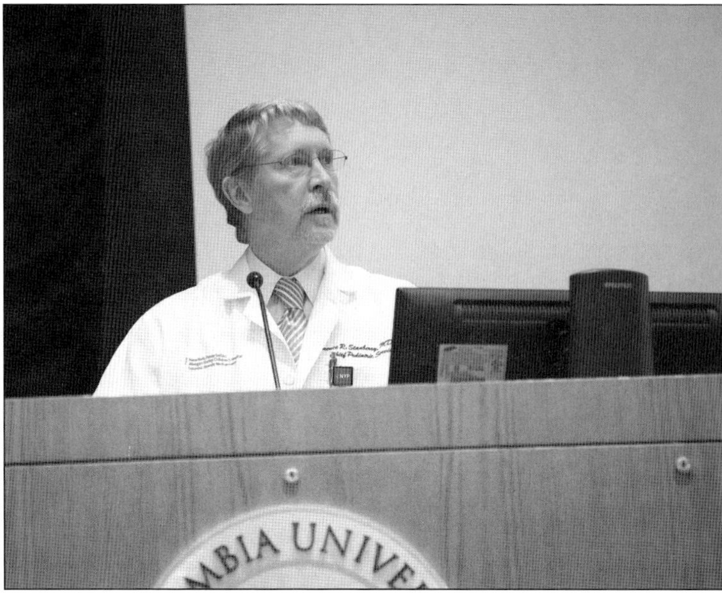

Steve Miller Day honors the life and legacy of Dr. Miller, former director of the pediatric emergency department, with a day of learning. Dr. Miller was tragically killed in a 2004 plane crash. Pictured at the podium during the 2015 event is Lawrence Stanberry, chair of the department of pediatrics at Columbia University Irving Medical Center, College of Physicians and Surgeons of Columbia University. (Photograph by Michael DeVito.)

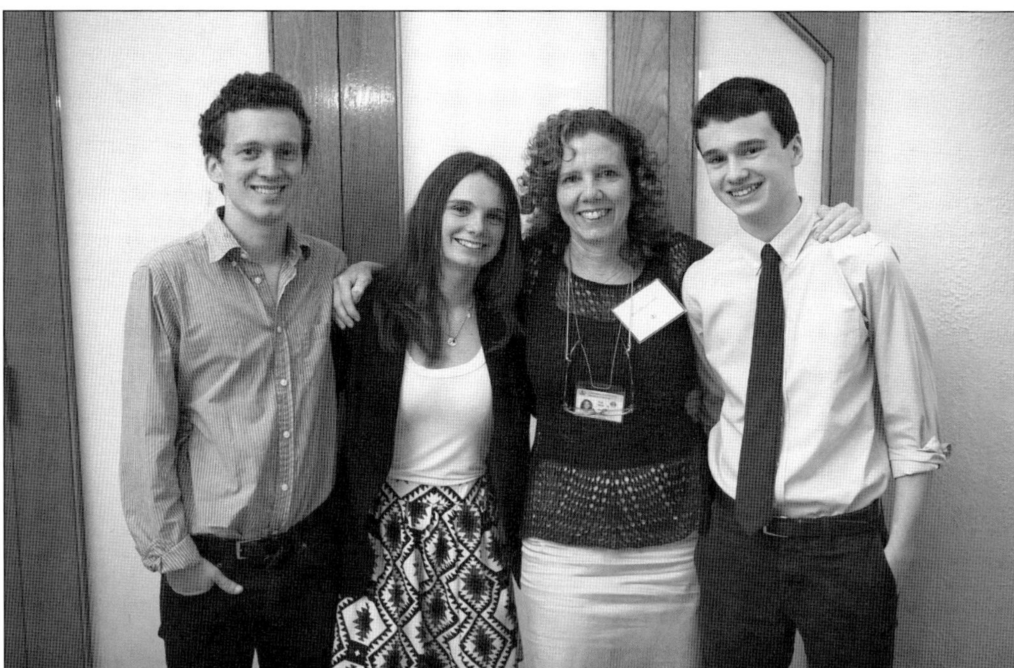

The celebration of the annual Steve Miller Day of learning provides visitors, residents, faculty, and staff with an opportunity to share in the humanism and memory of Dr. Miller. Pictured from left to right is the family of Steve Miller: Jesse Miller, Maya Miller, Dr. Dodi Meyer (Miller's widow and director of community pediatrics), and Nico Miller. (Photograph by Michael DeVito.)

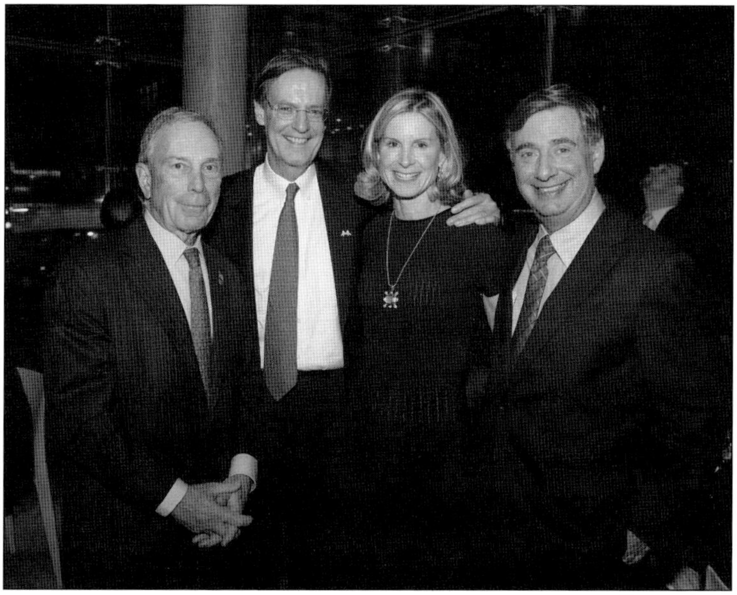

The Weinberg Family Cerebral Palsy Center was officially launched in 2013 thanks to lead gifts from Debby and Peter A. Weinberg along with several of their family members and friends. Pictured at the inaugural event in January 2013 to celebrate the opening of the center, from left to right, are New York City mayor Michael Bloomberg, Peter A. and Debby Weinberg, and Dr. Lee Goldman, dean of Columbia University's medical school.

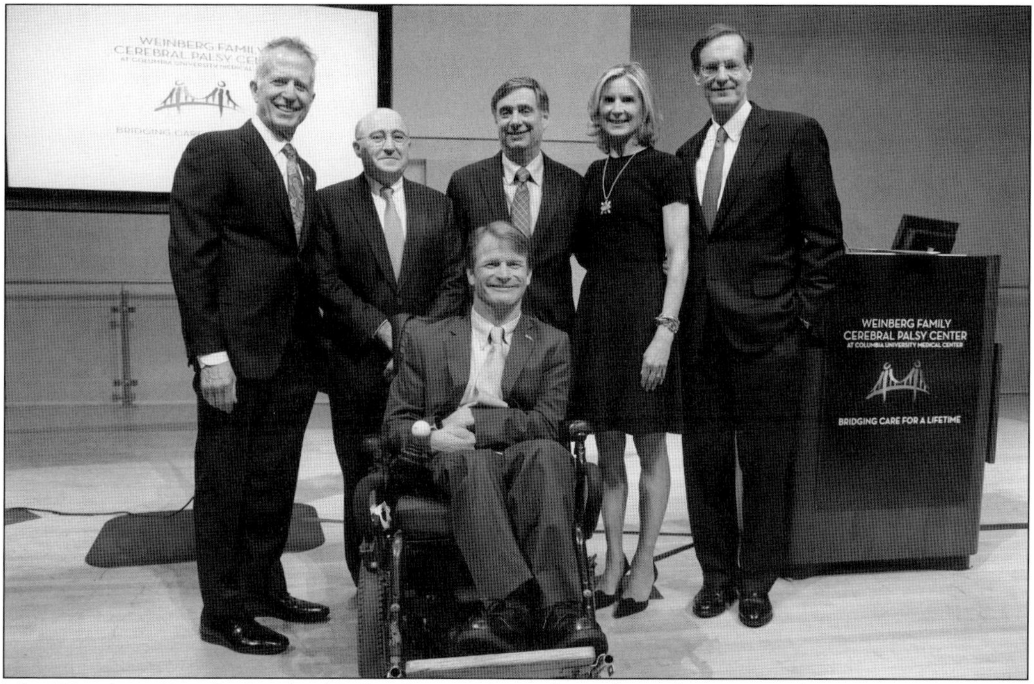

The Weinberg Family Cerebral Palsy Center, through its clinical services, education, and research programs, creates lifelong comprehensive care for those living with cerebral palsy. Pictured at the opening event in January 2013, from left to right, are founding executive director David P. Roye Jr.; Louis U. Bigliani, chair of the department of orthopedic surgery; Stephen Wampler; medical school dean Lee Goldman; Debby Weinberg; and Peter A. Weinberg. (Photograph by Michael DeVito.)

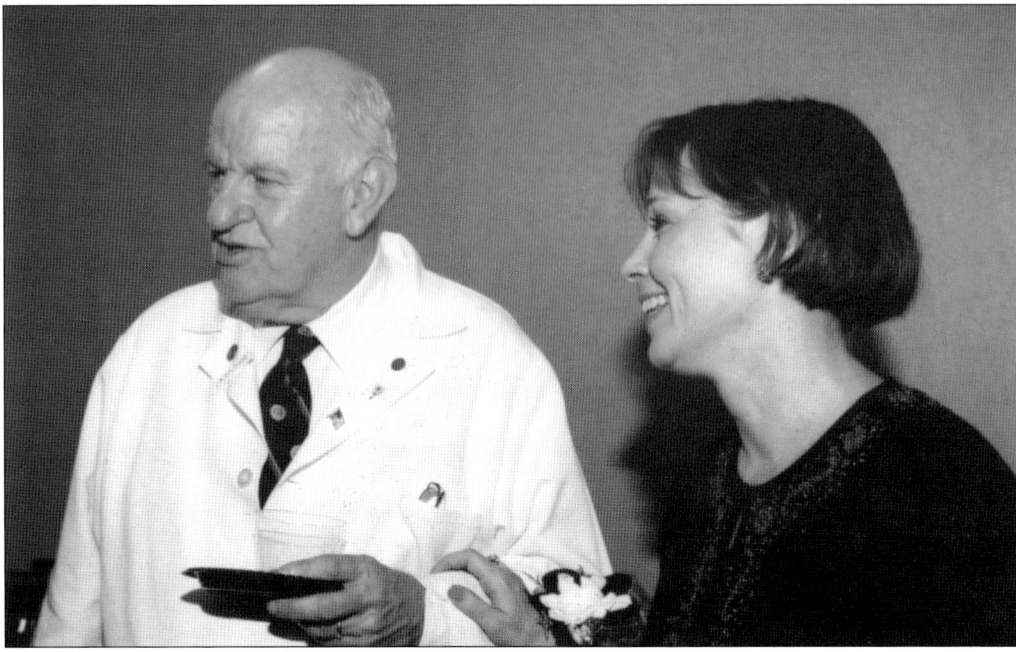

Dr. John M. Driscoll is seen here with Claire Pace at the annual fundraising luncheon on November 11, 2001. Pace, in honor of her son Adrian who was born with congenital heart disease, used her personal experience to connect with other parents and families dealing with their children's heart surgeries by hosting a weekly elegant English tea to provide an island of respite. (Photograph by Janet Charles.)

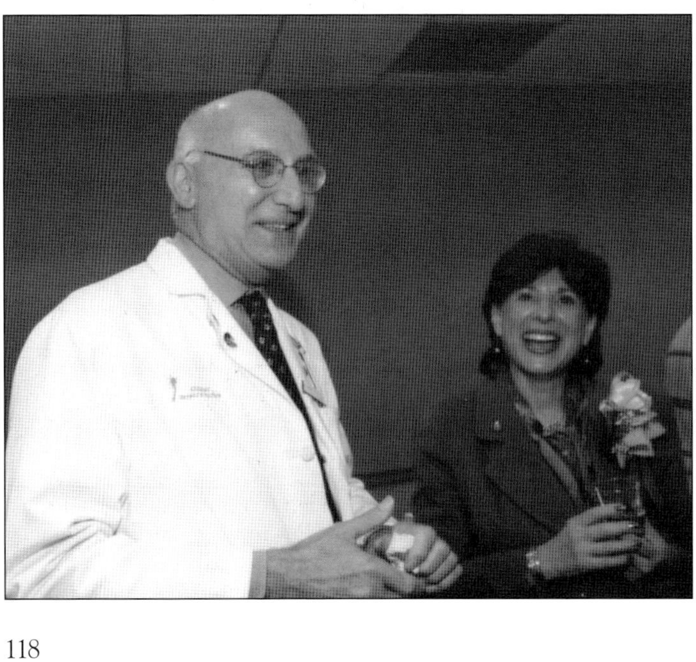

R. Peter Altman poses with Claire Pace at the annual luncheon on November 11, 2001. Dr. Altman came to Columbia University in 1980 as professor and surgeon-in-chief at Babies Hospital, a position he held for 19 years. His contributions include the surgical treatment of pediatric extrahepatic biliary disease and the Altman classification system for sacrococcygeal teratoma. He was president of the American Pediatric Surgical Association in 2002–2003. (Photograph by Janet Charles.)

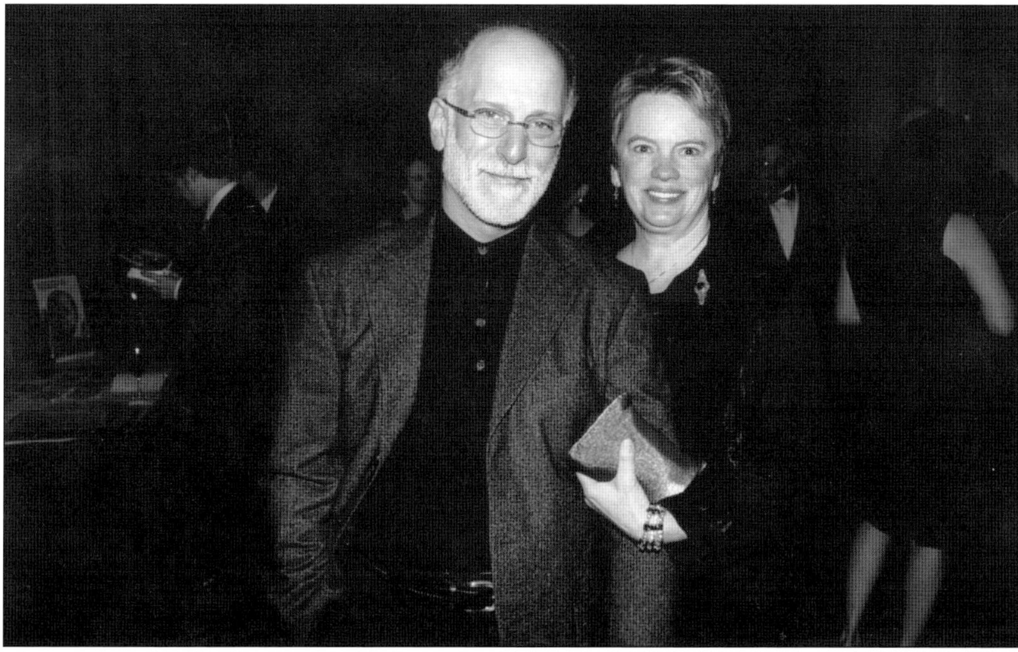

Physicians, staff, and colleagues enjoy one another's company at Friends and Family Day on December 3, 2003. Pictured are Dr. Charlie Stolar and his wife, Carolyn. Stolar was professor and director of pediatric surgery and surgeon-in-chief at Babies Hospital. He was instrumental in the development of ECMO, extracorporeal membrane oxygenation, which pumps and oxygenates a patient's blood outside the body, allowing the heart and lungs to rest. (Photograph by Marie Wallace.)

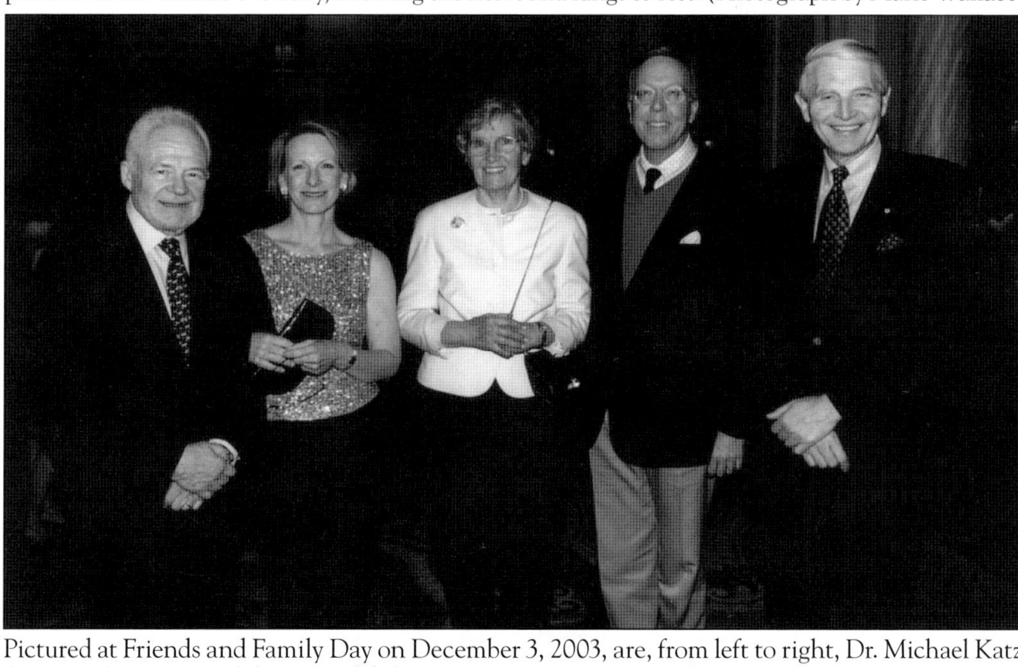

Pictured at Friends and Family Day on December 3, 2003, are, from left to right, Dr. Michael Katz, former Babies Hospital director and chair of pediatrics, and his wife, Robin; Dorothy Truman, wife of Dr. John Truman; Dr. Stephen W. Nicholas, pediatrician and dean of admissions at Columbia's medical school; and Dr. John Truman, vice chair of pediatrics. (Photograph by Marie Wallace.)

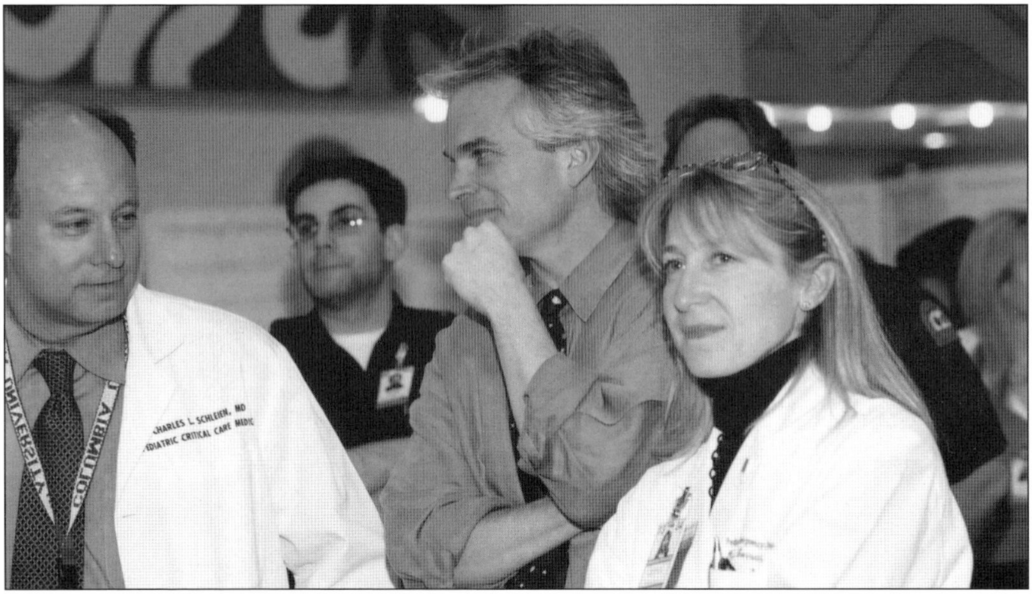

Friends and colleagues gather at Friends and Family Day on December 3, 2003. Pictured from left to right are Dr. Charles Schleien, director of critical care and pediatrician in charge of the intensive care unit; Dr. Steven Miller, humanist in medicine and director of the pediatric emergency department; and Dr. Meridith Sonnett, associate director of the pediatric emergency department. (Photograph by Marie Wallace.)

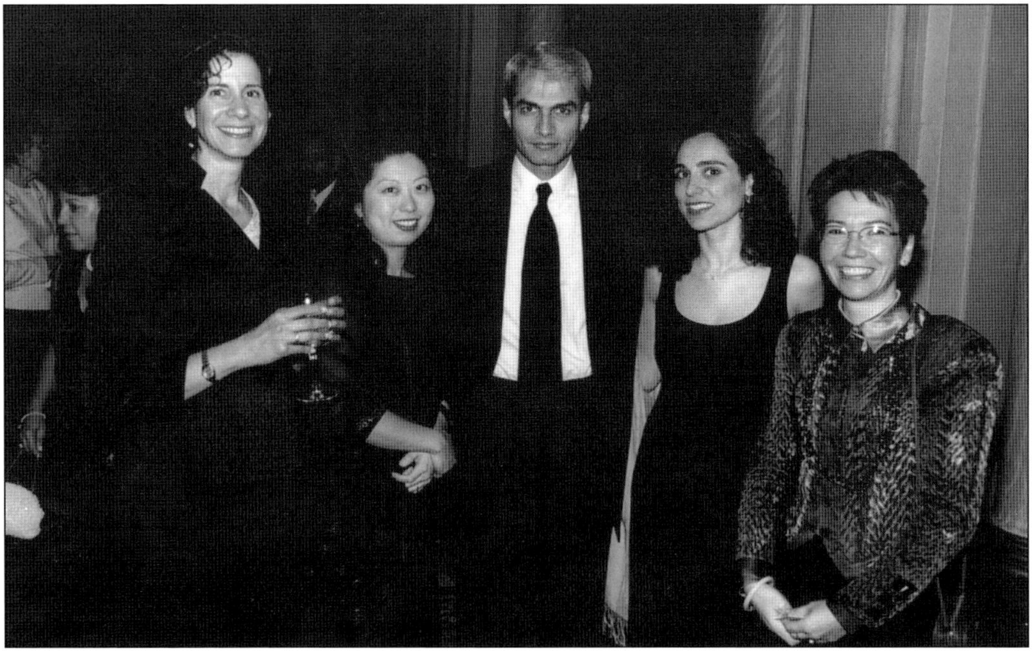

This image was also captured on Friends and Family Day, December 3, 2003. From left to right are Lisa Saiman, MD, member of the division of pediatric infectious disease and hospital epidemiologist; unidentified; Sujit Sheth, MD, member of the division of pediatric hematology; unidentified; and Betsy Wedemeyer, MD, member of the division of general pediatrics and director of the pediatric residency program at Morgan Stanley Children's Hospital. (Photograph by Marie Wallace.)

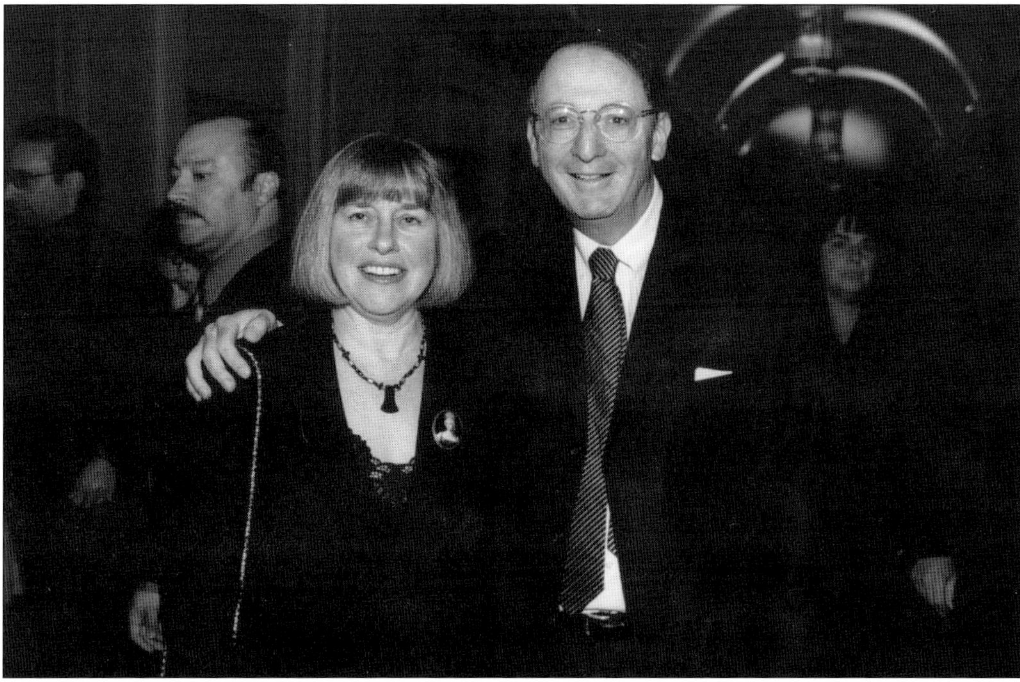

Rich Polin, MD, and his wife, Helene, celebrate Friends and Family Day, December 3, 2003. Dr. Polin is the William T. Speck Professor, director of neonatology, and pediatrician-in-chief of the nurseries at Morgan Stanley Children's Hospital. He is the editor and author of *Fetal and Neonatal Physiology* and *Secrets in Neonatology*. (Photograph by Marie Wallace.)

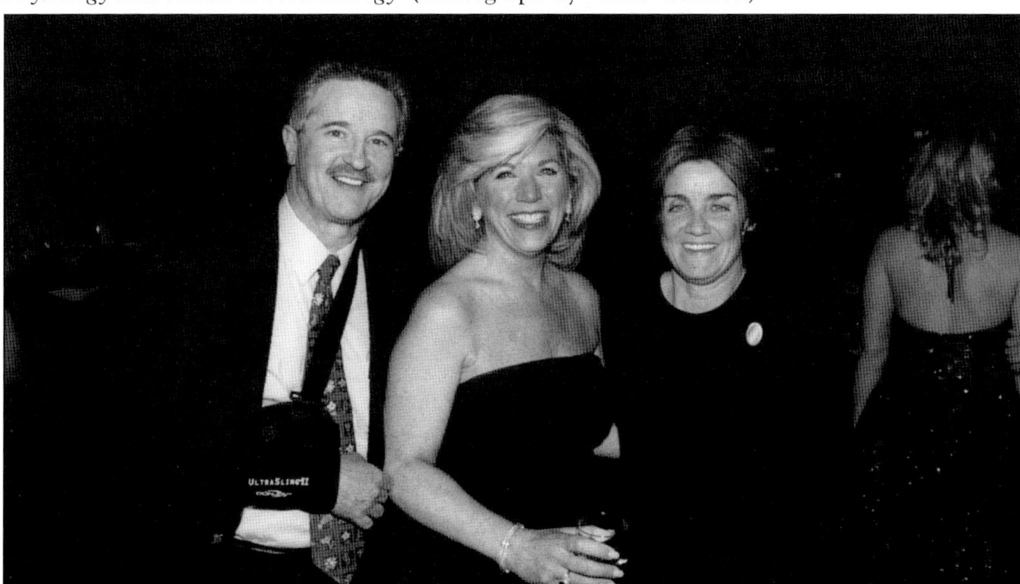

Friends and colleagues gather at Friends and Family Day, December 3, 2003. From left to right are Dr. Max Gomez, medicine and science writer and on-air reporter for WCBS; Cynthia Sparer, senior vice president and executive director of the Morgan Stanley Children's Hospital; and Peggy Quinn, RN, MPH, associate director of nursing and director of nursing quality at Morgan Stanley Children's Hospital. (Photograph by Marie Wallace.)

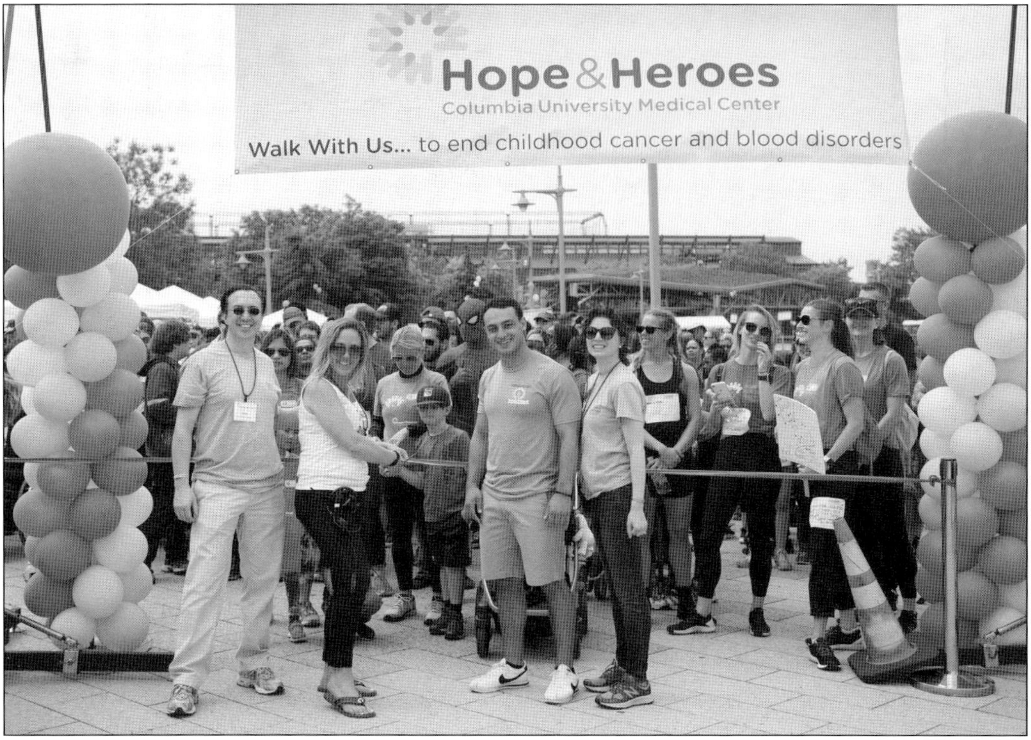
Hope&Heroes
Columbia University Medical Center
Walk With Us... to end childhood cancer and blood disorders

Michael Weiner, MD, established the Hope & Heroes Children's Cancer Fund in 1996 to raise much-needed philanthropic dollars to support oncology patients, research, education, and cutting-edge therapies. The fund is a 501(c)(3) with an independent board of directors. Pictured above is the start of the annual fundraising walkathon in May 2019 showing, from left to right, Bob Bombersbach, executive director of the charity; Patty Cavallo and Avery Hoffman, cochairs of the walkathon; and Katie Leiby, events coordinator. The photograph below, from the 2019 annual dinner gala, shows, from left to right, Peter Cieszko, Hope & Heroes board member; Robert Kapito, chairman of the Hope & Heroes board; and Michael Weiner, founder of Hope & Heroes and director of pediatric oncology at Morgan Stanley Children's Hospital. (Both photographs by Jenny Gorman.)

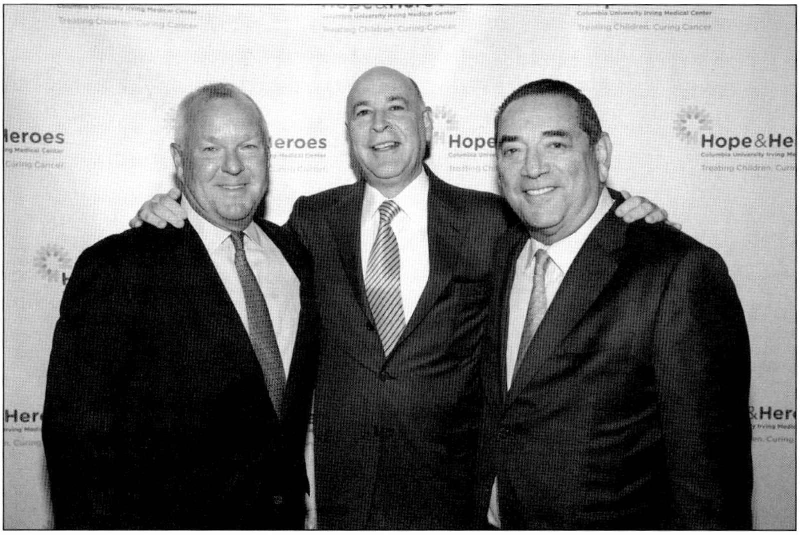

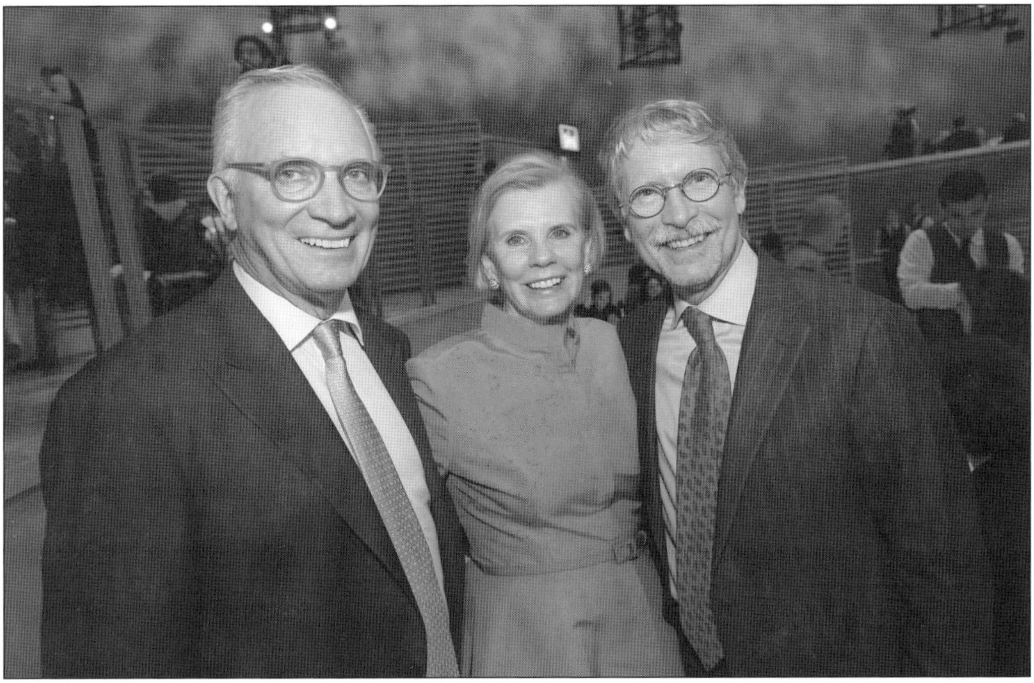

The Children's Board at Columbia was created to provide advice and philanthropic resources for important pediatric programs and research. The Fourth Annual Children's Gala was held on May 17, 2017, at Jazz at Lincoln Center. Pictured from left to right are Kevin Kennedy; Karen Kennedy, MD, founder and chair of the Children's Board; and Lawrence Stanberry, MD, PhD, chair of the department of pediatrics. (Photograph by Jenny Gorman and John Calabrese.)

The Fifth Annual Children's Gala was held on Monday, May 14, 2018, at Jazz at Lincoln Center. Seen on the left is Lee Goldman, dean of the Vagelos College of Physicians and Surgeons of Columbia University, and on the right is Jordan Orange, MD, PhD, chair of the department of pediatrics. (Photograph by Jenny Gorman and John Calabrese.)

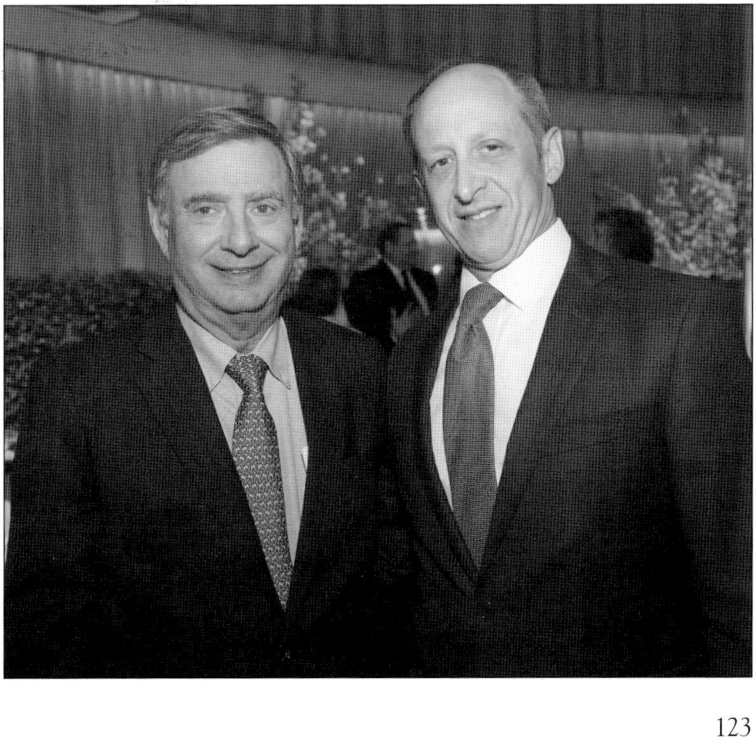

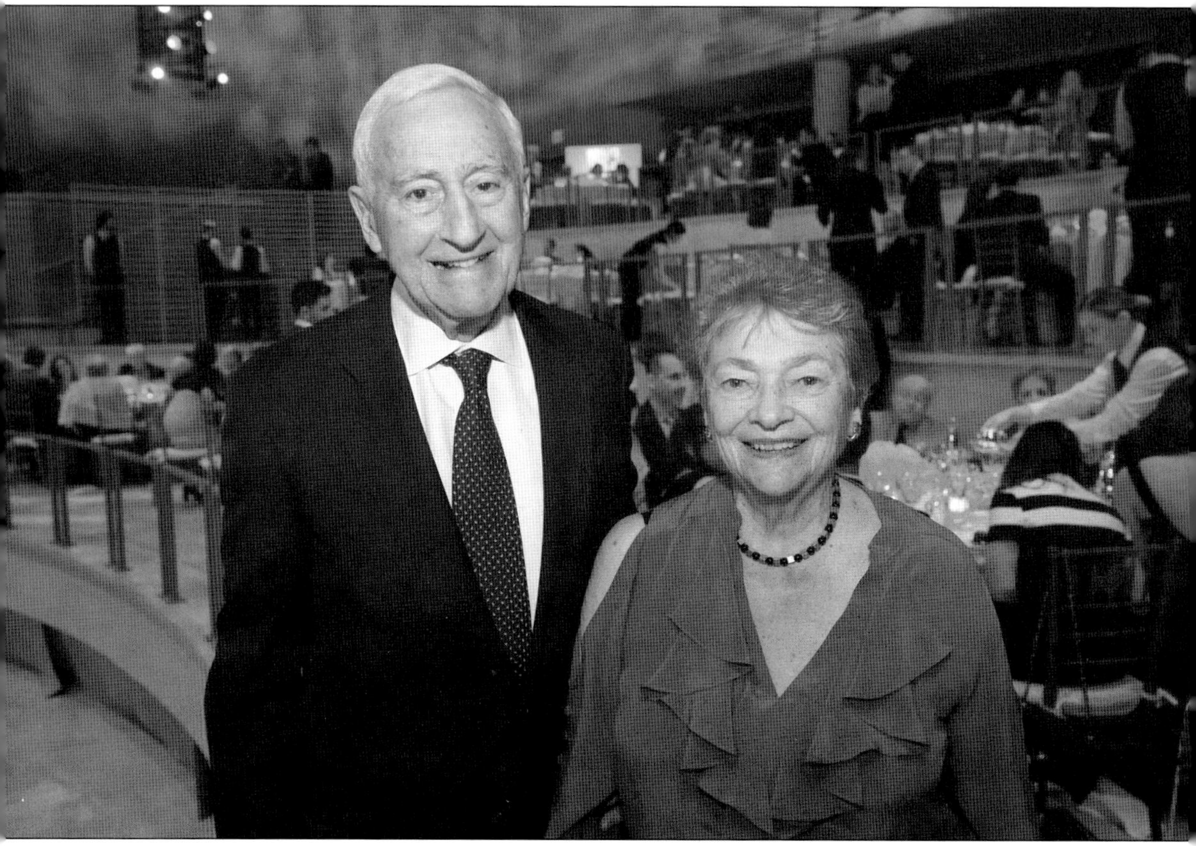

Pictured here are Roy Vagelos and his wife, Diana. Dr. Vagelos, a son of Greek immigrants, attended the University of Pennsylvania for undergraduate studies and received his medical degree from Columbia University College of Physicians and Surgeons in 1954. After a brief period at the National Institutes of Health, the Massachusetts General Hospital, and the Washington University School of Medicine, he joined Merck, Sharp & Dohme Research Laboratories in Rahway, New Jersey, where he became president and chief executive officer. Roy and Diana Vagelos have been major donors to Columbia's school of medicine, and in their honor, in 2017 it was renamed the Roy and Diana Vagelos College of Physicians and Surgeons of Columbia University. Dr. Vagelos has been elected to the American Academy of Arts and Sciences, the US National Academy of Sciences, and the American Philosophical Society. (Photograph by Jenny Gorman and John Calabrese.)

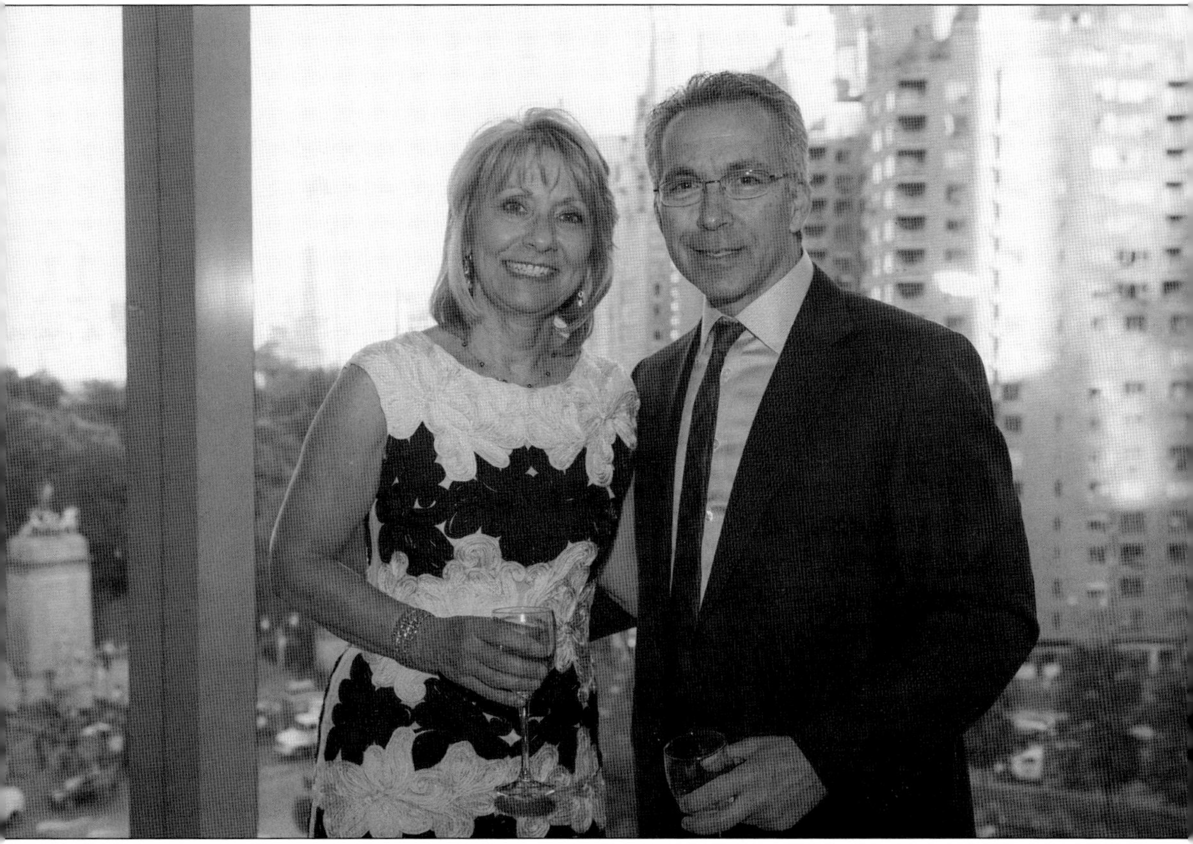

Steve Stylianos and his wife, Joann, enjoy the annual Children's Gala, held on May 17, 2017, at Jazz at Lincoln Center. A graduate of Rutgers University and the New York University School of Medicine, Dr. Stylianos completed his general surgical training at the Babies Hospital, Columbia-Presbyterian Medical Center. He completed a two-year fellowship at the Kiwanis Pediatric Trauma Institute in Boston before formal pediatric surgery training at Boston Children's Hospital. Dr. Stylianos joined the faculty of the Columbia University College of Physicians and Surgeons and the Babies Hospital of New York in 1992. Stylianos directed the multidisciplinary teams of physicians and nurses who separated five sets of conjoined twins. He has served as chairman of the trauma committee, 1997–2002, and as a member of the board of directors and treasurer of the American Pediatric Surgical Association. Dr. Stylianos is the Rudolph N. Schullinger Professor of Surgery and Pediatrics and chief of the division of pediatric surgery. (Photograph by Jenny Gorman and John Calabrese.)

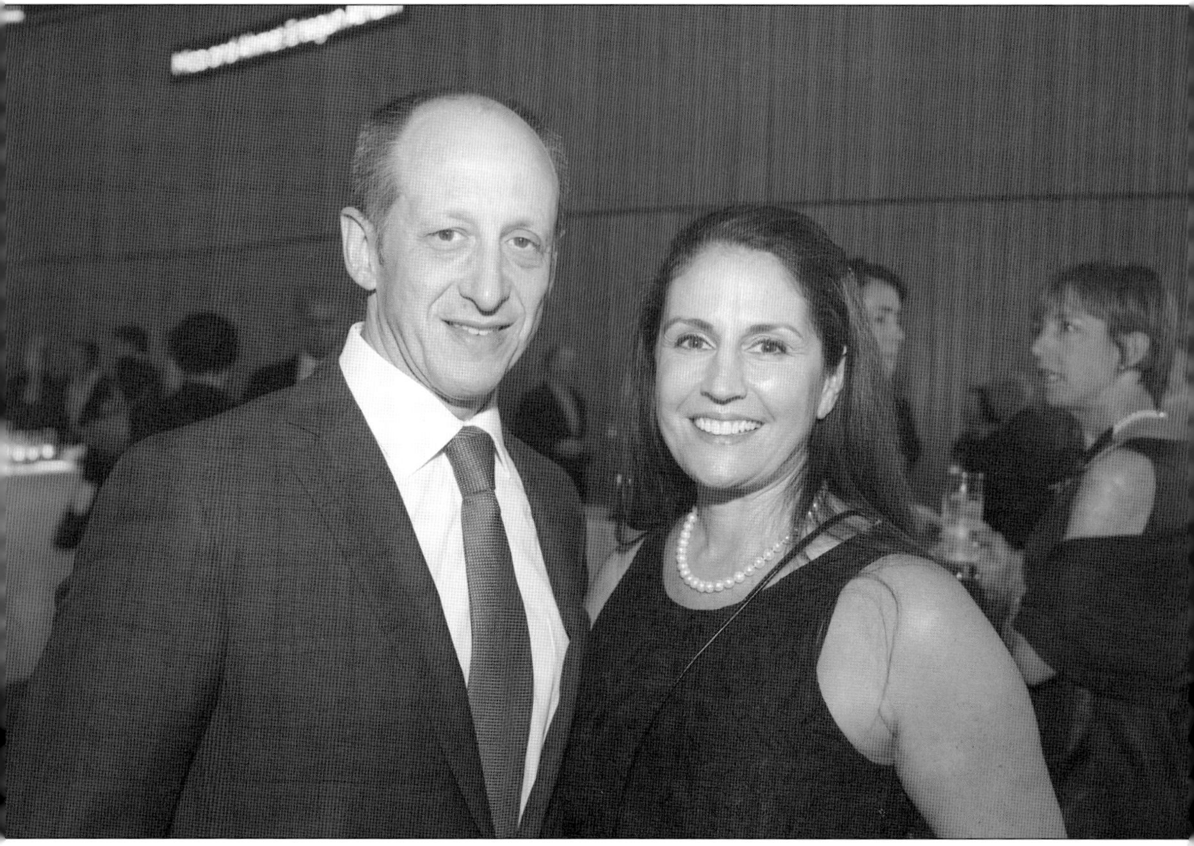

Jordan Scott Orange, MD, PhD, seen here with his wife, Katie, in 2019, was appointed the Reuben S. Carpentier Professor and chairman of the department of pediatrics at Columbia's Vagelos College of Physicians and Surgeons and pediatrician-in-chief of the NewYork-Presbyterian/Morgan Stanley Children's Hospital in 2018. He received his bachelor's, doctoral, and medical degrees from Brown University and went on to residency training at Children's Hospital of Philadelphia and a clinical fellowship and postdoctoral research fellowship at Boston Children's Hospital. He held faculty positions at the Children's Hospital of Philadelphia and Texas Children's Hospital at Baylor. He is an international leader in pediatric primary immunodeficiency and the immunobiology of human natural killer cells. In his research, Dr. Orange combines novel disease discovery with basic cell research to translate underlying biological mechanisms of disease into clinical applications. Dr. Orange is a member of the American Society for Clinical Investigation and the American Pediatric Society and was a recipient of the E. Mead Johnson Award for research accomplishment in pediatrics from the Society for Pediatric Research. He was recently elected a fellow of the National Academy of Medicine. (Photograph by Jenny Gorman and John Calabrese.)

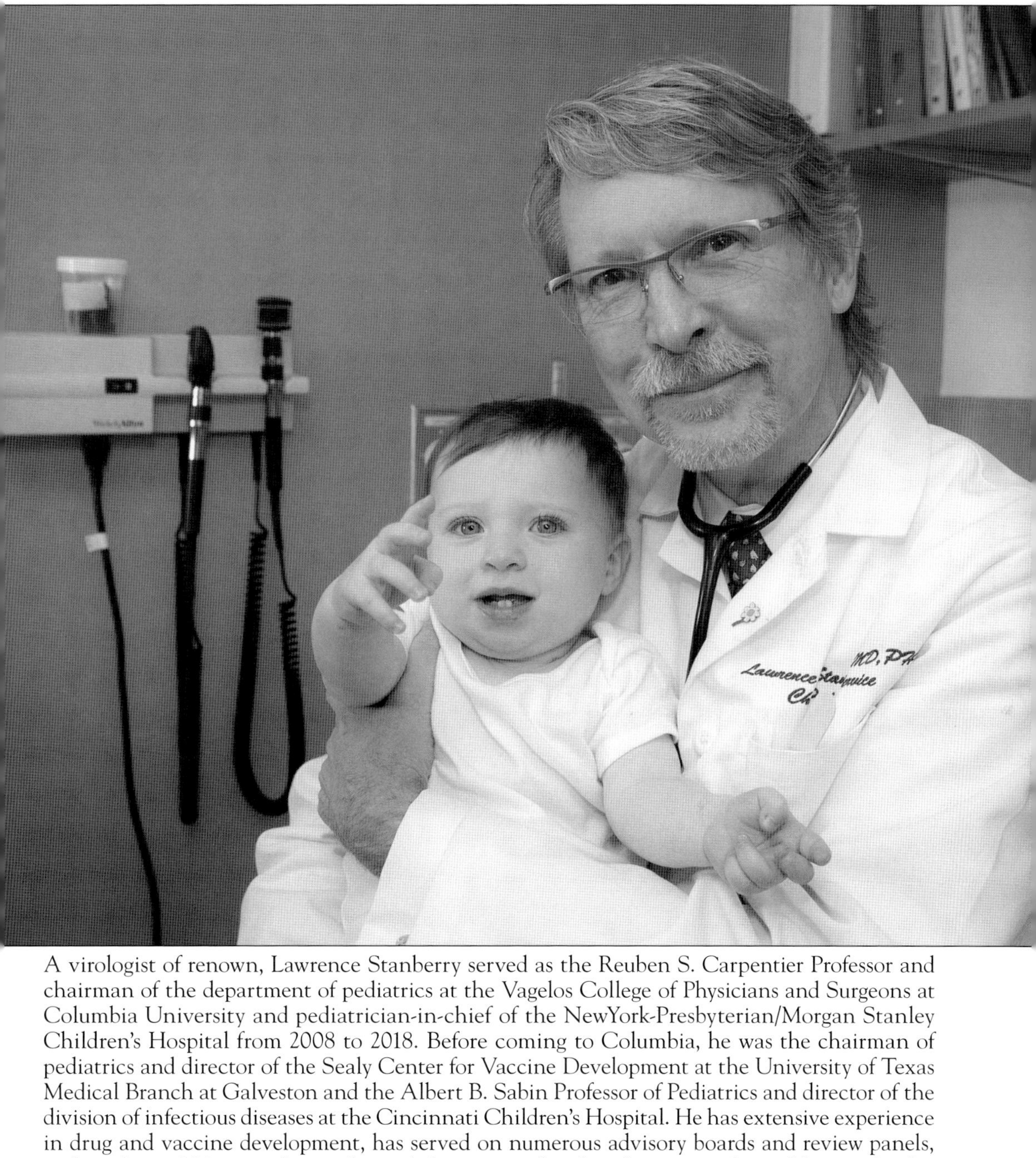

A virologist of renown, Lawrence Stanberry served as the Reuben S. Carpentier Professor and chairman of the department of pediatrics at the Vagelos College of Physicians and Surgeons at Columbia University and pediatrician-in-chief of the NewYork-Presbyterian/Morgan Stanley Children's Hospital from 2008 to 2018. Before coming to Columbia, he was the chairman of pediatrics and director of the Sealy Center for Vaccine Development at the University of Texas Medical Branch at Galveston and the Albert B. Sabin Professor of Pediatrics and director of the division of infectious diseases at the Cincinnati Children's Hospital. He has extensive experience in drug and vaccine development, has served on numerous advisory boards and review panels, authored over 200 scientific articles and chapters, and is the editor or coeditor of five textbooks, including *Understanding Modern Vaccines* and *Viral Infections of Humans: Epidemiology and Control.* Dr. Stanberry is currently the associate dean and director for international programs at Columbia. His current work focuses on the preparedness of children's hospitals globally to prevent, detect, and respond to infections with pandemic potential. (Photograph by Amelia Panico.)

Consistent with our mission to preserve history on a local level, this book was printed in South Carolina on American-made paper and manufactured entirely in the United States. Products carrying the accredited Forest Stewardship Council (FSC) label are printed on 100 percent FSC-certified paper.

MADE IN THE USA